Traditional Chinese Medical Therapies

Hand Therapy:
Traditional Chinese Remedies

Compiled by Wang Sheng and Wang Weidong

FOREIGN LANGUAGES PRESS

First Edition   1997
Second Printing   1998

Translated by Wang Tai

ISBN-7-119-01901-5

© Foreign Languages Press, Beijing, China, 1997

Published by Foreign Languages Press
24 Baiwanzhuang Road, Beijing 100037, China

Distributed by China International Book Trading Corporation
35 Chegongzhuang Xilu, Beijing 100044, China
P.O.Box 399, Beijing, China

Printed in the People's Republic of China

FOREWORD

As an important component of traditional Chinese medicine, the therapies applied to the hand—hand therapy—are a group of unique therapeutic methods developed by medical specialists and common people in China through their medical practice, productive activity, and daily lives for hundreds of years.

According to the meridian theory of traditional Chinese medicine, the hand is closely connected through meridians with the skin, blood vessels, muscles, ligaments, bones, and internal organs of the body. Pathological disease in patients is reflected on their hands; and the stimulating and therapeutic effects of massage, acupuncture, herbal bath, and *qigong* can be transmitted through meridians to adjust and stimulate potential energy, immunity, resistance to disease, and physical well-being to maintain health and prolong life.

Hand therapy can be easily practiced and widely applied to treat many diseases, often with good therapeutic results, and without toxic side effects. These therapies have found favor among vast numbers of patients over the years. To help foreign readers understand, learn, and practice this unique hand therapy, the compilers reviewed a large amount of ancient and modern medical literature in China, and have collected the useful experience of specialists in this field to systematically present the sum of this beneficial knowledge.

CONTENTS

Chapter 1
INTRODUCTION

Hand therapy for the treatment of general diseases of the body is a group of very convenient therapeutic methods applying different types of stimulation at various specific parts of the hand to promote circulation of *qi* and blood through meridians. This therapy can improve life quality, maintain health, and prevent and cure many diseases. The specific parts of hand are classified as the regular, extra, and special acupoints of the hand, homographic reflective points, and a group of points beside the second metacarpal bone. Stimulating methods include massage, acupuncture, herbal bath, and *qigong* applied at hand. Although these methods vary, they are all applied to the hand, and are, therefore, all included under the general name of hand therapy.

I. Origin and Development of Hand Therapy

Hand therapy is a component of traditional Chinese medicine.

According to the history of medicine, the origin of hand therapy was much earlier than that of medicinal therapy. In primitive times, human beings lived in caves in the open country and they would automatically rub their hands to promote blood circulation to prevent frostbite during the cold winter season; and rub or press painful areas to relieve their sufferings, resolve swelling and correct functional imbalances. Because pressure applied at Hegu (LI 4) acupoint of the hand could relieve toothache, people gradually found that stimulation applied at certain specific parts of the hand by pressing, rubbing, twisting and kneading, or by some tool, could produce certain therapeutic effects. This was none other than the primitive form of hand therapy.

In the ancient classic medical book the *Yellow Emperor's Internal Classic*, which was published during the Spring and Autumn and Warring States periods (770-221 B.C.), there are descriptions of the use of meridians and acupoints of the hand to diagnose and treat diseases. This shows that hand therapy is at least more than 2,000 years old.

Along with the increase of clinical practice and the accumulation of medical knowledge, and especially with the development of acupuncture, *tuina* (traditional Chinese massage), *qigong* and the use of medicinal herbs, the contents of hand therapy have greatly been enriched and expanded.

The theoretical basis of hand therapy is the meridian theory. Together with meridian theory and acupuncture practice, the functions of meridians and regular, extra, and special acupoints of the hand have been summarized and discussed in Chinese medical literature throughout different historical eras. The modern homographic theory of biology also substantiates the theories of hand therapy.

The development of *tuina* has also added to the contents of hand massage. In the *Yellow Emperor's Internal Classic*, the earliest tools of Chinese massage, such as round-tip needles and spoon needles, were first mentioned. The first book on *tuina* was published in the Qin and Han dynasties (221 B.C.-A.D. 220) 2,000 years ago. Since then, *tuina* has had a continuous development and has been spread to Japan, Korea, and India.

As an exercise for the body and mind, Chinese *qigong* exercises also have a long history and substantial content, and were developed by the Chinese people through the activities of their daily life to maintain health and treat diseases. *Qigong* of the hand is a modification of general *qigong* exercises.

The treatment of diseases using medicinal herbs is another important branch of traditional Chinese medicine. Herbal bath for the hand is an external therapy used in traditional Chinese medicine.

The hand is also a window revealing information about diseases and a mirror reflecting the health of the body. Nowadays, dermatoglyphics as a new branch of medical science has endowed traditional Chinese hand therapy with a new significance. The nail, fingerprints, and palm prints have great value for clinical practice.

As a component part of the body, the hand is closely connected with other parts of the body in a common internal environment. So the hand can be used to diagnose and treat diseases. These days people are more aware of the importance of maintaining their health. Therefore, hand therapy has become more and more welcomed by vast numbers of patients because it is safe, reliable, and easy to perform for both early diagnosis and treatment. In hand therapy, its non-medicinal nature and the use of natural herbs also have attracted the attention of more and more people in the world.

II. Hand Therapy Indications, Characteristics, and Precautions

1. Indications:

1) Painful diseases: Neurotic headache, trigeminal neuralgia, toothache, angina pectoris, chest pain, intercostal neuralgia, neuralgia sciatica, and abdominal pain.

2) Chronic diseases: Bronchitis, peptic stomach ulcer, chronic gastroenteritis, diarrhea, diabetes mellitus, rheumatism, soft tissue injury, chronic nephritis, hemiplegia, arthritis, and muscular strain of the waist.

3) Functional diseases: Irregular menstruation, dysmenorrhea, functional disturbance of vegetative nervous system, intestinal paralysis, and stomach spasms.

4) Neurological diseases: Neurasthenia, spasm of facial muscles, facial palsy, and neurotic deafness.

5) Inflammatory diseases: Tonsillitis, pharyngitis, stomatitis,

rhinitis, bronchitis, periarthritis of shoulder, cholecystitis, nephritis, and arthritis.

6) Acute diseases: High fever with convulsions, acute angina pectoris, acute attack of epilepsy, acute larygopharyngitis, acute conjunctivitis, and acute gastritis.

2. Characteristics:

1) Holistic principles in the treatment of disease are followed. This includes treating internal diseases with external therapy and treating general diseases with local therapy.

2) Hand therapy is a simple treatment with numerous indications, including common internal diseases, surgical problems, and gynaecological, pediatric, and ENT disorders.

3) This treatment is cheap, convenient and safe.

4) It can be used to treat diseases as well as improve the health of normal people.

5) It can be done by the patients themselves for early diagnosis and treatment.

6) It can produce good therapeutic results without harmful side effect.

7) The techniques of hand therapy can be widely popularized for broad application.

3. Precautions:

1) Care must be taken in treating pregnant women at early and later stages of pregnancy.

2) It must be used with care in potential surgical conditions such as acute appendicitis with indication of surgical intervention.

3) Hand therapy is prohibited for patients with necrotic, infectious, or pyogenic skin lesions of the hand.

Chapter 2
COMMON ACUPOINTS FOR HAND THERAPY

The acupoints for hand therapy include the regular and extra acupoints on the hand. The acupoints on the forearm are also used in hand therapy because they are exposed and convenient to locate for application of acupuncture (the acupoints marked with an asterisk (*) are located on the hand).

1. Chize (LU 5, on hand Taiyin lung meridian)

Location: With elbow slightly flexed, it is on the cubital crease and on the radial border of tendon of brachial biceps muscle (Fig. 1).

Function: To suppress adverse ascent of lung *qi*, tone lung *yin*, and moisten the lung.

Indications: Cough, asthma, hemoptysis, sore throat, chest distension, acute mastitis, arm and elbow pain, vomiting, and diarrhea.

Acupuncture: Vertical insertion of needle for 1.6 cm, or bleeding therapy with three-edged needle; and moxibustion is permissible.

2. Kongzui (LU 6, on hand Taiyin lung meridian)

Location: With arm extended and palm supine, it is on the connecting line between Chize (LU 5) and Taiyuan (LU 9) and 23.3 cm from Taiyuan (Fig. 1).

Function: To suppress adverse ascent of lung *qi*, clear blood heat, and stop bleeding.

Indications: Cough, asthma, hemoptysis, sore throat, aphonia, hemorrhoids, and arm and elbow pain.

Acupuncture: Vertical insertion of needle for 1.6-3.3 cm; and moxibustion is permissible.

3. Lieque (LU 7, on hand Taiyin lung meridian)

Location: It is proximal to radial styloid process and 5 cm proximal to carpal crease (Fig. 1).

Function: To expel pathogen from lungs and adjust Renmai (conceptional vessel).

Indications: Cough, asthma, sore throat, hemiplegia, deviation of mouth and eye, migraine, stiff neck, toothache, and hotness in palm.

Acupuncture: Oblique insertion of needle toward elbow for 0.7 cm; and moxibustion is permissible.

4. Jingqu (LU 8, on hand Taiyin lung meridian)

Location: With palm supine, it is 3.3 cm proximal to carpal crease and in a depression between radial styloid process and radial artery (Fig. 1).

Function: To control cough and asthma and adjust breath.

Indications: Cough, asthma, sore throat, pain and distension

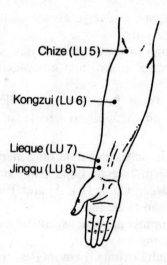

Chize (LU 5)

Kongzui (LU 6)

Lieque (LU 7)
Jingqu (LU 8)

Fig. 1

in chest, and hotness in palm.

Acupuncture: Vertical insertion of needle for 1 cm; and moxibustion is permissible.

5. Taiyuan* (LU 9, on hand Taiyin lung meridian)

Location: With palm supine, it is on carpal crease and in a depression on the radial side of radial artery (Fig. 2).

Function: To control cough, resolve phlegm, improve body resistance, and expel pathogens.

Indications: Cough, asthma, hemoptysis, pain and distension of chest, sore throat, vomiting, abdominal distension, irregular pulse, and hand and wrist pain.

Acupuncture: Vertical insertion of needle for 1 cm; and moxibustion is permissible.

6. Yuji* (LU 10, on hand Taiyin lung meridian)

Location: With palm supine, it is proximal to the first metacarpophalangeal joint, at the midpoint of metacarpal bone and on the dorsopalmar boundary (Fig. 2).

Function: To clear heat in lungs, relieve stagnation in throat, and clear heat in blood.

Indications: Cough, hemoptysis, sore throat, elbow spasm, and hotness in palm.

Acupuncture: Vertical insertion of needle for 1.6-3.3 cm; and moxibustion is permissible.

7. Shaoshang* (LU 11, on hand Taiyin lung meridian).

Location: On the radial side of thumb and 0.3 cm from corner of nail (Fig. 2).

Function: To clear heat, open sense organ orifices, restore *yang*, revive critical patients, relieve stagnation in throat, and control convulsion.

Indications: Cough, asthma, sore throat, madness, epilepsy, stroke with coma, febrile diseases, and convulsion in children.

Acupuncture: Horizontal insertion of needle toward wrist for 0.6 cm or bleeding therapy with three-edged needle; and moxibustion is permissible.

8. Shangyang* (LI 1, hand Yangming large intestine meridian)

Location: On the radial side of index finger and 0.3 cm from the corner of nail (Fig. 3).

Function: To clear heat, resolve swelling, open sense organ orifices, and refresh the mind.

Indications: Sore throat, swelling of jaw, toothache, deafness, tinnitus, cough, asthma, stroke with coma, and shoulder pain.

Acupuncture: Upward oblique insertion of needle for 0.6 cm or bleeding therapy with three-edged needle; and moxibustion is permissible.

9. Erjian* (LI 2, on hand Yangming large intestine meridian)

Location: With hand slightly clenched, it is on the radial side of second metacarpophalangeal joint and distal to it, and on the dorsopalmar boundary of hand (Fig. 3).

Function: To clear heat and resolve swelling.

Indications: Sore throat, swelling of jaw, nasal bleeding, toothache, eye pain, deviation of mouth and eye, body heat, and shoulder pain.

Acupuncture: Vertical insertion of needle for 0.6 cm; and moxibustion is permissible.

10. Sanjian* (LI 3, on hand Yangming large intestine meridian)

Location: With hand slightly clenched, it is on the radial side

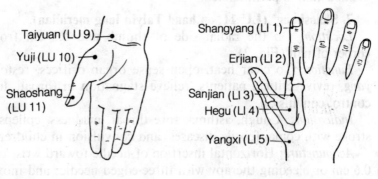

Taiyuan (LU 9)
Yuji (LU 10)
Shaoshang (LU 11)
Shangyang (LI 1)
Erjian (LI 2)
Sanjian (LI 3)
Hegu (LI 4)
Yangxi (LI 5)

Fig. 2   Fig. 3

of index finger and proximal to second metacarpophalangeal joint and capitulum of second metacarpal bone (Fig. 3).

Function: To clear heat, resolve swelling, relieve fullness, and stop diarrhea.

Acupuncture: Vertical insertion of needle for 1 cm; and moxibustion is permissible.

11. Hegu* (LI 4, on hand Yangming large intestine meridian)

Location: Between the first and second metacarpal bone and at the midpoint of second metacarpal bone (Fig. 3).

Function: To clear heat, treat exterior syndrome, and improve vision and hearing.

Indications: Headache, dizziness, toothache, eye pain, sore throat, swelling of face, deviation of mouth and eye, diseases of nose and ear, fever, hemiplegia, finger spasms, arm pain, amenorrhea, late delivery of baby, skin rashes, and diseases of stomach and intestines.

Acupuncture: Vertical insertion of needle for 1.6-3.3 cm; and moxibustion is permissible.

12. Yangxi* (LI 5, on hand Yangming large intestine meridian)

Location: On the radial side of dorsum of wrist and in a depression between tendons of long and short extensor muscles of thumb (Fig. 3).

Function: To clear heat, tranquilize the mind, improve vision, and remove stagnation in throat.

Indications: Headache, sore throat, red eyes, deafness, tinnitus, toothache, arm and wrist pain, epilepsy, and madness.

Acupuncture: Vertical insertion of needle for 1.3 cm; and moxibustion is permissible.

13. Pianli (LI 6, on hand Yangming large intestine meridian)

Location: On the connecting line between Yangxi (LI 5) and Quchi (LI 11) acupoints and 10 cm from Yangxi (Fig. 4).

Function: To improve vision and hearing.

Indications: Nasal bleeding, red eyes, tinnitus, deafness, deviation of mouth and eye, sore throat, edema and pain in

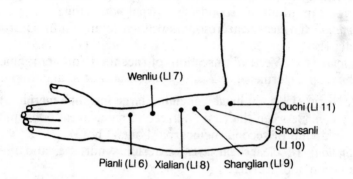

Fig. 4

shoulder, arm, elbow, and wrist.

Acupuncture: Oblique insertion of needle for 1 cm; and moxibustion is permissible.

14. Wenliu (LI 7, on hand Yangming large intestine meridian)

Location: On the connecting line between Yangxi (LI 5) and Quchi (LI 11) acupoints and 16.6 cm from Yangxi (Fig. 4).

Function: To clear heat, resolve swelling, tranquillize the mind, and promote transportation in organs.

Indications: Headache, facial swelling, nose bleed, sore throat, pain in shoulder and back, epilepsy, and madness.

Acupuncture: Vertical insertion of needle for 1.6 cm; and moxibustion is permissible.

15. Xialian (LI 8, on hand Yangming large intestine meridian)

Location: On the connecting line between Yangxi (LI 5) and Quchi (LI 11) acupoints and 1.3 cm from Quchi (Fig. 4).

Function: To adjust *qi* and promote transportation in organs.

Indications: Headache, dizziness, abdominal pain, acute mastitis, and pain in elbow and arm.

Acupuncture: Vertical insertion of needle for 1.6 cm; and moxibustion is permissible.

16. Shanglian (LI 9, on hand Yangming large intestine meridian)

Location: On the connecting line between Yangxi (LI 5) and Quchi (LI 11) acupoints and 10 cm from Quchi (Fig. 4).

Function: To adjust *qi* and promote transportation in organs.

Indications: Headache, pain in shoulder and arm, abdominal pain, diarrhea, and hemiplegia.

Acupuncture: Vertical insertion of needle for 1.6-3.3 cm; and moxibustion is permissible.

17. Shousanli (LI 10, on hand Yangming large intestine meridian)

Location: On the connecting line between Yangxi (LI 5) and Quchi (LI 11) acupoints and 6.7 cm from Quchi (Fig. 4).

Function: To clear heat, improve vision, adjust *qi*, and promote transportation in organs.

Indications: Abdominal distension, diarrhea, eye diseases, toothache, hemiplegia, and hand, arm, and elbow pain.

Acupuncture: Vertical insertion of needle for 1.6-3.3 cm; and moxibustion is permissible.

18. Quchi (LI 11, on hand Yangming large intestine meridian)

Location: With elbow flexed, it is in a depression on the radial end of cubital crease (Fig. 4).

Function: To expel wind pathogen, control itching, clear heat, and resolve swelling.

Indications: Febrile diseases, sore throat, toothache, eye pain, skin rashes, skin sores, scabies, diseases of stomach and intestine, epilepsy, madness, disturbance of menstruation, paralysis of upper limb, and shoulder and arm pain.

Acupuncture: Vertical insertion of needle for 3.3-5 cm; and moxibustion is permissible.

19. Shaohai (HT 3, on hand Shaoyin heart meridian)

Location: With elbow flexed, it is in a depression on the ulnar end of cubital crease (Fig. 5).

Function: To tranquilize the mind.

Indications: Heart pain, epilepsy, madness, tuberculosis of cervical lymph nodes, hand tremors and spasms, and pain in armpit.

Acupuncture: Vertical insertion of needle for 1.6-3.3 cm; and moxibustion is permissible.

20. Lingdao (HT 4, on hand Shaoyin heart meridian)

Location: With hand supine, it is on the radial border of ulnar flexor muscle of wrist and 5 cm proximal to carpal crease (Fig. 5).

Function: To expand chest and adjust *qi*.

Indications: Heart pain and palpitations, dizziness, vertigo, unreasonable crying and laughing, stiff tongue, aphasia, and wrist and arm spasms.

Acupuncture: Vertical insertion of needle for 1 cm; and moxibustion is permissible.

21. Tongli (HT 5, on hand Shaoyin heart meridian)

Location: With hand supine, it is on the radial border of ulnar flexor muscle of wrist and 3.3 cm proximal to carpal

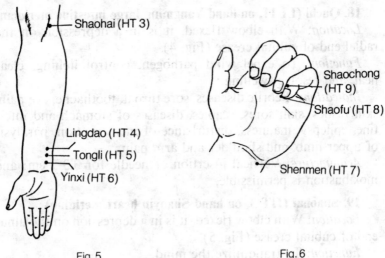

Shaohai (HT 3)

Lingdao (HT 4)
Tongli (HT 5)
Yinxi (HT 6)

Shaochong (HT 9)
Shaofu (HT 8)
Shenmen (HT 7)

Fig. 5   Fig. 6

crease (Fig. 5).

Function: To tranquilize the mind, tone *yin*, and clear heart heat.

Indications: Heart palpitations, stiff tongue, aphasia, profuse uterine bleeding, headache, vertigo, and pain on medial and posterior side of shoulder, elbow, and arm.

Acupuncture: Vertical insertion of needle for 1 cm; and moxibustion is permissible.

22. Yinxi (HT 6, on hand Shaoyin heart meridian)

Location: With hand supine, it is on the radial border of ulnar flexor muscle of wrist and 1.6 cm proximal to carpal crease (Fig. 5).

Function: To tranquilize the mind and clear heat in the blood.

Indications: Heart pain and palpitations, night sweating, aphasia, and hematemesis.

Acupuncture: Vertical insertion of needle for 1 cm; and moxibustion is permissible.

23. Shenmen* (HT 7, on hand Shaoyin heart meridian)

Location: On the carpal crease and on the radial border of ulnar flexor muscle of wrist (Fig. 6).

Function: To improve the body's resistance, expel pathogens, and tranquilize the mind.

Indications: Heart pain and palpitations, insomnia, poor memory, unreasonable crying and laughing, epilepsy, madness, headache, vertigo, and hotness in palm.

Acupuncture: Vertical insertion of needle for 1 cm; and moxibustion is permissible.

24. Shaofu* (HT 8, on hand Shaoyin heart meridian)

Location: It is proximal to the fourth and fifth metacarpophalangeal joints; with the hand supine and fingers flexed, it is in the depression between the tips of ring and little fingers (Fig. 6).

Function: To clear heat of the heart and tranquilize the mind.

Indications: Heart pain and palpitations, unreasonable crying and laughing, incontinence of urine, pain in external genitalia, and prolapse of uterus.

Acupuncture: Vertical insertion of needle for 1 cm; and moxibustion is permissible.

25. Shaochong* (HT 9, hand Shaoyin heart meridian)

Location: On the radial side of little finger and 0.3 cm from the corner of nail (Fig. 6).

Function: To clear heat, control convulsions, and tranquilize and refresh the mind.

Indications: Heart pain and palpitations, pain in chest and flanks, coma, epilepsy, madness, febrile diseases, and pain in medial and posterior side of arm.

Acupuncture: Oblique insertion of needle for 0.3 cm or bleeding therapy with three-edged needle; and moxibustion is permissible.

26. Shaoze* (SI 1, on hand Taiyang small intestine meridian)

Location: On the ulnar side of little finger and 0.3 cm from the corner of nail (Fig. 7).

Function: To increase body fluid, promote discharge of milk, clear heat, and facilitate discharge through orifices.

Indications: Febrile diseases, coma, oligogalactia, acute mas-

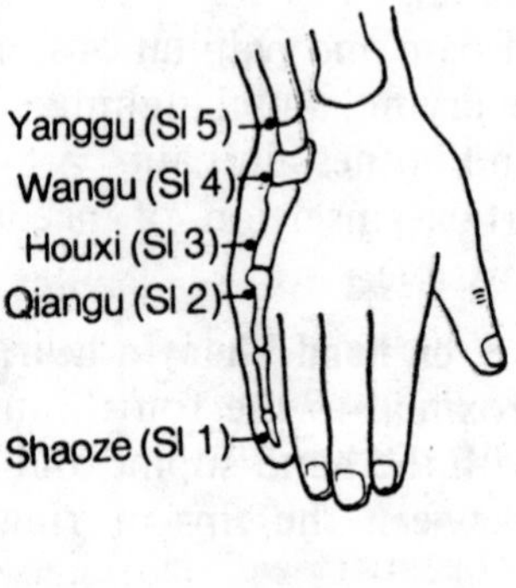

Yanggu (SI 5)
Wangu (SI 4)
Houxi (SI 3)
Qiangu (SI 2)
Shaoze (SI 1)

Fig. 7

titis, headache, sore throat, and pain in lateral and posterior side of shoulder and arm.

Acupuncture: Oblique insertion of needle for 0.3 cm or bleeding therapy; and moxibustion is permissible.

27. Qiangu* (SI 2, on hand Taiyang small intestine meridian)

Location: Distal to the fifth metacarpophalangeal joint and on its ulnar side. As the hand is clenched, it is at the end of a crease distal to that metacarpophalangeal joint and on the dorsopalmar boundary of hand.

Function: To disperse liver *qi*, clear heart heat, and improve vision and hearing.

Indications: Neck pain, numbness and pain in elbow, arm and fingers, epilepsy, madness, sore throat, and oligogalactia.

Acupuncture: Vertical insertion of needle for 1 cm; and moxibustion is permissible.

28. Houxi* (SI 3, on hand Taiyang small intestine meridian)

Location: It is proximal to the fifth metacarpophalangeal joint, on its ulnar side and on the posterior border of the fifth metacarpal bone. With the hand clenched, it is at the end of a crease proximal to that joint (Fig. 7).

Function: To clear heart heat, relieve depression, and control malaria with fever.

Indications: Headache, stiff neck, deafness, febrile diseases, night sweating, malaria, epilepsy, madness, spasms of elbow, arm and little finger, and scabies.

Acupuncture: Vertical insertion for 1.6-3.3 cm; and moxibustion is permissible.

29. Wangu* (SI 4, on hand Taiyang small intestine meridian)

Location: On the distal border of triangular bone and on the dorsopalmar boundary of hand (Fig. 7).

Function: To increase body fluids, relieve thirst, promote the discharge of bile, and reduce jaundice.

Indications: Headache, stiff neck, jaundice, chest pain, thirst, finger spasms, and arm pain.

Acupuncture: Vertical insertion of needle for 1 cm; and moxibustion is permissible.

30. Yanggu* (SI 5, on hand Taiyang small intestine meridian)
Location: Between the pisiform bone and ulnar styloid process, and on the dorsopalmar boundary (Fig. 7).
Function: To clear heart heat, tranquilize the mind, and improve vision and hearing.
Indications: Vertigo, red eyes, ear diseases, toothache, scabies, swelling of neck and jaw, and pain in lateral side of arm, hand and wrist.
Acupuncture: Vertical insertion of needle for 1 cm; and moxibustion is permissible.

31. Yanglao (SI 6, on hand Taiyang small intestine meridian)
Location: With the palm prone, it is on the eminence of ulnar styloid process (Fig. 8).
Function: To increase body fluids for nourishing muscles, and clear head heat for improving vision.
Indications: Acute lumbago, blurred vision, and pain in shoulder, back, elbow and arm.
Acupuncture: With palm on chest, the needle is obliquely inserted toward elbow for 1.6-2.6 cm; and moxibustion is permissible.

32. Zhizheng (SI 7, on hand Taiyang small intestine meridian)
Location: On the connecting line between Yanggu (SI 5) and Xiaohai (SI 8) and 16.6 cm proximal to wrist (Fig. 8).
Function: To disperse liver *qi*, tranquilize the mind, clear heat, and treat exterior syndromes.
Indications: Stiff neck, headache, madness with unreasonable crying and laughing, diabetes mellitus, scabies, elbow spasm and finger pain.
Acupuncture: Vertical insertion of needle for 1.3 cm; and moxibustion is permissible.

33. Xiaohai (SI 8, on hand Taiyang small intestine meridian)
Location: With elbow flexed, it is between the olecranon and

medial epicondyle of humerus (Fig. 8).

Function: To disperse liver *qi*, tranquilize the mind, clear heat, and resolve swelling.

Indications: Swelling of cheek, headache, dizziness, ear diseases, epilepsy, madness, and pain in lateral and posterior side of shoulder and arm.

Acupuncture: Vertical insertion of needle for 1 cm; and moxibustion is permissible.

34. Quze (PC 3, on hand Jueyin pericardium meridian)

Location: With hand supine and elbow slightly flexed, it is on the cubital crease and on the ulnar border of brachial biceps muscle (Fig. 9).

Function: To clear heart heat, control pain, adjust the stomach, and suppress adverse ascent of *qi*.

Indications: Heart pain and palpitations, cough, stomachache, vomiting, and elbow and arm pain.

Acupuncture: Vertical insertion of needle for 1.6-3.3 cm or bleeding therapy with three-edged needle; and moxibustion is permissible.

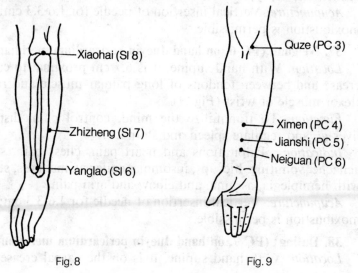

Xiaohai (SI 8)

Quze (PC 3)

Zhizheng (SI 7)

Ximen (PC 4)
Jianshi (PC 5)
Neiguan (PC 6)

Yanglao (SI 6)

Fig. 8   Fig. 9

35. Ximen (PC 4, on hand Jueyin pericardium meridian)

Location: With hand supine, it is on the connecting line between Quze (PC 3) and Daling (PC 7) acupoints and 16.6 cm from Daling, and between the tendons of long palmar muscle and radial flexor muscle of wrist (Fig. 9).

Function: To clear heart heat, control cough, clear blood heat, and stop bleeding.

Indications: Pain and palpitations of heart, anxiety, hemoptysis, hematemesis, epilepsy, and scabies.

Acupuncture: Vertical insertion of needle for 1.6-3.3 cm; and moxibustion is permissible.

36. Jianshi (PC 5, on hand Jueyin pericardium meridian)

Location: With hand supine, it is 10 cm proximal to the carpal crease and between the tendons of long palmar muscle and radial flexor muscle of wrist (Fig. 9).

Function: To expand chest, relieve depression, tranquilize the mind and suppress adverse ascent of *qi*.

Indications: Heart pain and palpitations, vomiting, stomachache, epilepsy, madness, elbow spasms and arm pain.

Acupuncture: Vertical insertion of needle for 1.6-3.3 cm; and moxibustion is permissible.

37. Neiguan (PC 6, on hand Jueyin pericardium meridian)

Location: With hand supine, it is 6.7 cm proximal to carpal crease and between tendons of long palmar muscle and radial flexor muscle of wrist (Fig. 9).

Function: To tranquilize the mind, control pain, disperse liver *qi*, and regulate spleen and stomach.

Indications: Palpitations and heart pain, chest pain, stomachache, vomiting, hiccups, insomnia, epilepsy, madness, stroke with hemiplegia, asthma, and elbow and arm pain.

Acupuncture: Vertical insertion of needle for 1.6-3.3 cm; and moxibustion is permissible.

38. Daling* (PC 7, on hand Jueyin pericardium meridian)

Location: With hand supine, it is on the carpal crease and between tendons of long palmar muscle and radial flexor muscle of wrist (Fig. 10).

Function: To tranquilize the mind, expand chest, and regulate stomach.

Indications: Heart pain and palpitations, vomiting, stomachache, pain in chest and flanks, epilepsy, madness, and wrist pain.

Acupuncture: Vertical insertion of needle for 1.3 cm; and moxibustion is permissible.

39. Laogong* (PC 8, on hand Jueyin pericardium meridian)

Location: With fingers flexed and hand clenched, it is where the palm is touched by the tip of the middle finger. (Fig. 10).

Function: To clear heart heat, tranquilize the mind, reduce swelling, and stop itching.

Indications: Stroke with coma, heat stroke, heart pain, epilepsy, madness, aphtha, and a foul smell in the mouth.

Acupuncture: Vertical insertion of needle for 1.3 cm; and moxibustion is permissible.

40. Zhongchong* (PC 9, on hand Jueyin pericardium meridian)

Location: At the tip of middle finger (Fig. 10).

Function: To open sense organ orifices, restore consciousness, and clear heart heat.

Indications: Stroke with coma, stiff tongue, aphasia, convulsions in children, febrile diseases, and heat stroke.

Acupuncture: Superficial puncture of needle for 0.3 cm or bleeding therapy with three-edged needle.

41. Guanchong* (TE 1, on hand Shaoyang triple energizer meridian)

Location: On the ulnar side of ring finger and 0.3 cm from the corner of nail (Fig. 11).

Function: To clear heat, treat exterior syndrome, clear heart heat, and improve hearing.

Indications: Headache, red eyes, ear diseases, stiff tongue, and febrile diseases.

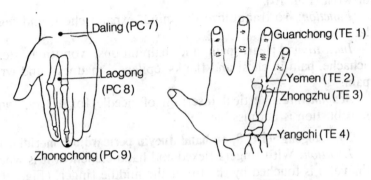

Fig. 10

Fig. 11

Acupuncture: Superficial insertion of needle for 0.3 cm or bleeding therapy with three-edged needle; and moxibustion is permissible.

42. Yemen* (TE 2, on hand Shaoyang triple energizer meridian)

Location: In the depression between and distal to the fourth and fifth metacarpophalangeal joints (Fig. 11).

Function: To clear heart heat, improve hearing, and regulate organ functions.

Indications: Headache, red eyes, ear diseases, and hand and arm pain.

Acupuncture: Vertical insertion of needle for 1 cm; and moxibustion is permissible.

43. Zhongzhu* (TE 3, on hand Shaoyang triple energizer meridian)

Location: Proximal to the fourth and fifth metacarpophalangeal joints and between the fourth and fifth metacarpal bones, 3.3 cm proximal to Yemen (TE 2) acupoint (Fig. 11).

Function: To clear heat, remove stagnation in throat, and improve vision and hearing.

Indications: Headache, vertigo, redness, swelling and pain in eyes, ear diseases, febrile diseases, and pain in shoulder, back, elbow and fingers.

Acupuncture: Vertical insertion of needle for 1.6 cm; and moxibustion is permissible.

44. Yangchi* (TE 4, on hand Shaoyang triple energizer meridian)

Location: With hand prone, it is on the dorsal crease of wrist and in the depression on the ulnar side of tendon of common extensor muscle of fingers (Fig. 11).

Function: To remove stagnation in throat, improve hearing, and regulate organ functions.

Indications: Ear diseases, diabetes mellitus, sore throat, and pain in shoulder, arm and wrist.

Acupuncture: Vertical insertion of needle for 1.3 cm; and moxibustion is permissible.

45. Waiguan (TE 5, on hand Shaoyang triple energizer meridian).

Location: Between radius and ulna bones and 6.7 cm proximal to Yangchi (TE 4) acupoint (Fig. 12).

Function: To treat exterior syndrome, clear heat, and improve hearing and vision.

Indications: Febrile diseases, cheek pains, ear diseases, red eyes, and pain in flanks, shoulder, back, elbow, arm, hand and fingers.

Acupuncture: Vertical insertion of needle for 1.6-3.3 cm; and moxibustion is permissible.

46. Zhigou (TE 6, on hand Shaoyang triple energizer meridian)

Location: Between radius and ulna bones and 10 cm proximal to Yangchi (SI 4) acupoint (Fig. 12).

Function: To clear heat, improve hearing, suppress adverse ascent of *qi*, and moisten intestines.

Indications: Ear diseases, constipation, pain in flanks, shoulder and back, and febrile diseases.

Acupuncture: Vertical insertion of needle for 3.3 cm; and

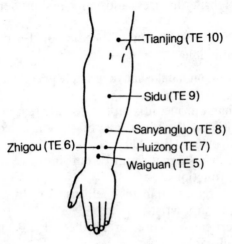

Fig. 12

moxibustion is permissible.

47. Huizong (TE 7, on hand Shaoyang triple energizer meridian)

Location: On the radial border of ulna bone, beside Zhigou (TE 6) acupoint and 10 cm proximal to Yangchi (TE 4) acupoint (Fig. 12).

Function: To improve hearing and control convulsions.

Indications: Deafness and pain in upper limb.

Acupuncture: Vertical insertion of needle for 1.6-3.3 cm; and moxibustion is permissible.

48. Sanyangluo (TE 8, on hand Shaoyang triple energizer meridian)

Location: Between radius and ulna bones and 13.3 cm proximal to Yangchi (TE 4) acupoint (Fig. 12).

Function: To improve hearing and remove stagnation in throat.

Indications: Sudden aphonia, deafness, toothache, and hand and arm pain.

Acupuncture: Vertical insertion of needle for 1.6-3.3 cm; and moxibustion is permissible.

49. Sidu (TE 9, on hand Shaoyang triple energizer meridian)

Location: Between radius and ulna bones and 16.6 cm distal to Zhoujian (EX-UE 1) acupoint (Fig. 12).

Function: To improve hearing and remove stagnation in throat.

Indications: Sudden aphonia, deafness, toothache, and forearm pain.

Acupuncture: Vertical insertion of needle for 1.6-3.3 cm; and moxibustion is permissible.

50. Tianjing (TE 10, on hand Shaoyang triple energizer meridian)

Location: With elbow flexed, it is in the depression proximal to olecranon (Fig. 12).

Function: To improve hearing, tranquilize the mind, adjust *qi*, and resolve phlegm.

Indications: Migraine, pain in neck, flank, ribs, shoulder and arm, ear diseases and tuberculosis of cervical lymph nodes.

Acupuncture: Vertical insertion of needle for 1.6-3.3 cm; and moxibustion is permissible.

51. Shixuan* (EX-UE 11, extra acupoint)

Location: On the tips of fingers and 0.3 cm from the free edge of nails (Fig. 13).

Function: To open sense organ orifices, restore consciousness, clear heat, and control convulsions.

Indications: Coma, heat stroke, febrile diseases, convulsions in children, sore throat, and numbness in fingertips.

Acupuncture: Vertical insertion of needle for 0.3 cm or bleeding therapy with three-edged needle.

52. Baxie* (EX-UE 9, extra acupoints)

Location: At the dorsal ends of creases between each pair of two neighboring fingers, with a total of eight acupoints on both hands (Fig. 14).

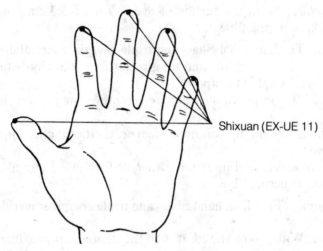

Shixuan (EX-UE 11)

Fig. 13

Function: To clear heat and reduce swelling.

Indications: Pain and swelling of hand dorsum, numbness in fingers, headache, stiff neck, toothache, and eye pain.

Acupuncture: Proximally oblique insertion of needle for 1.6 cm or bleeding therapy with three-edged needle; and moxibustion is permissible.

53. Zhongkui* (EX-UE 4, extra acupoint)

Location: With hand clenched, it is on the dorsal crease of proximal interphalangeal joint of middle finger (Fig. 14).

Function: To suppress adverse ascent of *qi* and regulate stomach.

Indications: Dysphagia, regurgitation of fluid, vomiting, hiccups, toothache, and nose bleed.

Acupuncture: Moxibustion.

54. Sifeng* (EX-UE 10, extra acupoints)

Location: With hand supine and fingers extended, they are at the midpoint of palmar creases of proximal interphalangeal joints of index, middle, ring, and little fingers (Fig. 15).

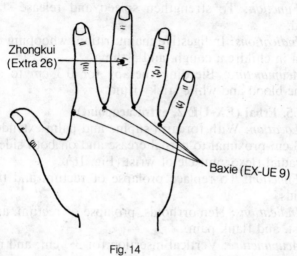

Zhongkui
(Extra 26)

Baxie (EX-UE 9)

Fig. 14

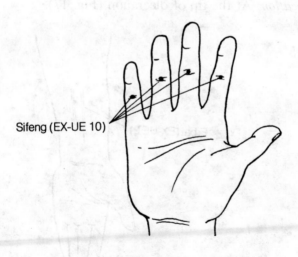

Sifeng (EX-UE 10)

Fig. 15

Function: To strengthen spleen and release stagnation of food.

Indications: Indigestive malnutrition, whooping cough, diarrhea in children, cough, and asthma.

Acupuncture: Bleeding therapy for 0.3 cm to squeeze out some blood and white sticky fluid.

55. Erbai (EX-UE 2, extra acupoint)

Location: With forearm supine and palm extended, they are 13.3 cm proximal to carpal crease and on both sides of tendon of radial flexor muscle of wrist (Fig. 16).

Function: To replace prolapse of rectum and treat hemorrhoids.

Indications: Hemorrhoids, prolapse of rectum, and forearm, chest, and flank pain.

Acupuncture: Vertical insertion for 3.3 cm; and moxibustion is permissible.

56. Zhoujian (EX-UE 1, extra acupoint)

Location: At the tip of olecranon (Fig. 17).

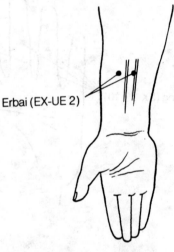

Erbai (EX-UE 2)

Fig. 16

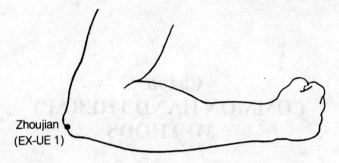

Fig. 17

Function: To resolve phlegm and swelling.

Indications: Tuberculosis, carbuncle, cellulitis, furuncle, and intestinal abscess.

Acupuncture: Moxibustion.

Chapter 3
COMMON HAND THERAPY METHODS

Although there are many therapeutic methods used for hand therapy, only the most common are discussed in this chapter. They include massage, acupuncture, hand bath, *qigong* and several miscellaneous methods including holding herbs, pressing and kneading the border of second metacarpal bone, arm swinging and other exercises.

I. Hand Therapy Massage

In hand therapy massage, stimulation is applied by hand to the regular and extra acupoints or reflective points and reflective areas closely related to various internal organs and tissues in the body. Particular maneuvers are employed to adjust their function, treat diseases, improve life quality, and maintain health. The basic maneuvers of massage include pressing, digit-pressing, kneading, pushing, pinching, twisting, rotating, pulling, rubbing, and grinding methods.

1. Pressing maneuver:

A vertical pressure is applied by the tip or pad of thumb at the acupoints, reflective areas, and reflective points (Fig. 18).

Indications: The pressing maneuver is usually applied at the acupoints on a flat area (such as thenar and hypothenar prominence) combined with a kneading maneuver to prevent and treat various chronic diseases and pains and maintain health.

Principle of manipulation: The thumb should be firmly applied on the skin to produce a steady and persistent pressure in a small area. The pressure should be gradually increased in intensity, and not suddenly applied with a violent action. The frequency and intensity of pressure should be even.

2. Digit-pressing maneuver:

A pressure is applied at the acupoints of the hand by the tip of thumb or middle finger; or by the lateral border of tip of little finger supported by thumb and ring finger; or by the knuckle of proximal interphalangeal joint of index finger (Fig. 19).

Indications: The digit-pressing maneuver is usually applied with a heavy pressure at acupoints in a fissure between bones, or in a limited area to treat acute or painful diseases.

Principle of manipulation: Compared with the pressing maneuver, this maneuver can produce a stronger stimulation in a smaller area. The pressure should be applied at an accurate location without any sliding movement. The intensity of pressure may vary over a wide range.

3. Kneading maneuver:

The pad of thumb or middle finger is placed at the acupoint of the hand to receive treatment, and the forearm is actively swung to and fro with the elbow as a fulcrum and the wrist, palm, and finger as a transmitter to produce a gentle rotating and kneading movement to the acupoint with the pad of finger (Fig. 20).

Indications: The kneading maneuver is usually applied at acupoints situated superficially over a broad area to produce an adjusting and toning effect for treatment of chronic, deficient, and wasting diseases as well as for maintenance of health and relief of local swelling and pain.

Principle of manipulation: The pressure applied by the kneading maneuver should be gentle and the movement of finger, hand and arm should be coordinated, rhythmic, and persistent for a longer period of time.

4. Pushing maneuver:

The single or multiple finger(s), root of palm, thenar or hypothenar prominence is used to produce an unidirectional

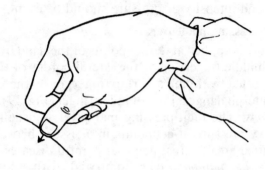

Fig. 18   Pressing maneuver

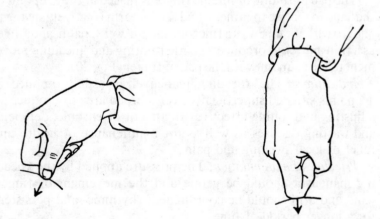

(1) Finger-pressing maneuver   (2) Knuckle-pressing maneuver

Fig. 19   Digit-pressing maneuver

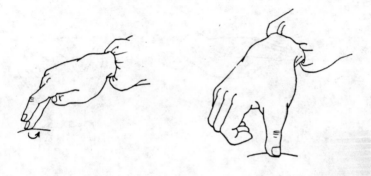

(1) Kneading with middle finger   (2) Kneading with thumb

Fig. 20 Kneading maneuver

linear pushing movement over certain parts of the hand (Fig. 21).

Indications: The pushing maneuver is usually applied along the longitudinal direction of the hand or over various sides of the fingers, and it may be followed by a rubbing maneuver to maintain health and treat chronic diseases, pain, and soreness due to soft tissue strain or diseases caused by deficiency and cold.

Principle of manipulation: To apply the pushing maneuver, the pushing force must be steady and strong enough, with the finger or palm placed firm on the skin of the hand. The pushing speed should be slow and even. The direction of the pushing maneuver is along the bones of the hand, and the force of the pushing maneuver may be freely adjusted, but it should be maintained at a fixed depth.

5. Pinching maneuver:

The free border or radial corner of the thumb nail or free border of the nails of other fingers is used to apply a vertical, heavy stimulation to the hand acupoints; or the free border of the thumb nail and the free border of the nails of other fingers

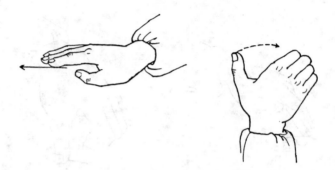

(1) Pushing with palm root   (2) Pushing with finger

Fig. 21 Pushing maneuver

are used to pinch the acupoint from both sides (Fig. 22).

Indications: The pinching maneuver is usually applied between metacarpal bones or between metacarpophalangeal joints together with pressing, kneading, and twisting maneuvers (or alternately applied) to treat acute or painful diseases, epilepsy, and neurasthenia.

Principle of manipulation: This is a maneuver designed to produce a heavy and deep stimulation and response. After the heavy and deep pinching manipulation is held for half a minute, gentle pressing and kneading maneuvers should follow for half a minute to relieve the discomfort produced by the pinching maneuver. This manipulation is repeated a second time. The pinching maneuver may be applied for a shorter duration and with a quicker rhythm. The nail must be steadily applied at the acupoint without any sliding movement to avoid causing injury to the skin.

6. Twisting maneuver:

The pads of thumb and index finger are used to hold and twist the injured finger back and forth to promote blood circulation through collaterals and stop pain (Fig. 23).

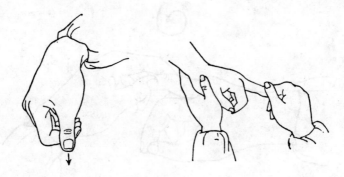

Fig. 22 Pinching maneuver   Fig. 23 Twisting maneuver

Indications: The twisting maneuver is usually applied to the small joints of the fingers, together with pinching and pushing maneuvers to treat chronic diseases and local discomforts, and to maintain health.

Principle of manipulation: The twisting maneuver should be applied gently without any sliding movement, or vigorously without any roughness. The quick rhythm and nimble application at thinner parts (like fingers) of the body are important characteristics of the twisting maneuver. Otherwise, the slow and forcible rotating movement applied to thicker parts of the body with opposite fingers is known as the kneading maneuver, rather than the twisting maneuver.

7. Rotating maneuver:

This is a manipulation to passively and evenly rotate finger and wrist joints for relaxing and adjusting joints and improving their movement (Fig. 24).

Indications: The rotating maneuver is usually applied to fingers and wrist for improving their active movement, slowing the aging process, curing diseases, maintaining the health of the hand, and treating chronic and senile diseases and local injuries.

Principle of manipulation: For convenient, safe and reliable application of this maneuver, it is best performed by both hands

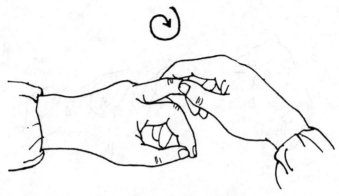

Fig. 24 Rotating maneuver

of the practitioner. One hand is used to fix the patient's hand, and the other is used to rotate the patient's finger or wrist. The force applied to rotate the finger or wrist should be balanced on both sides. Otherwise, they may be injured. Before rotating the finger or wrist, the pulling and twisting maneuvers should be applied first to relax the joints to avoid damaging them.

8. Pulling maneuver:

This is a manipulation used to apply extension and traction to one end of a joint, while another end is fixed. It is usually used to treat the joints of fingers and wrist to relax and increase their range of motion, improve general health, and slow the aging process (Fig. 25).

Indications: The pulling maneuver is usually applied to inter-phalangeal, metacarpophalangeal, and wrist joints to treat joint diseases of the hand and maintain the health of elderly people.

Principle of manipulation: The pulling maneuver should be nimbly and cooperatively performed by both hands of the practitioner with an adequate force and at an even speed, but without any roughness or violence. The pulling force should be exactly applied along the longitudinal axis of the joints without any angulation to avoid damaging the joint and ligament. The crackle of the joint caused by the pulling maneuver should not

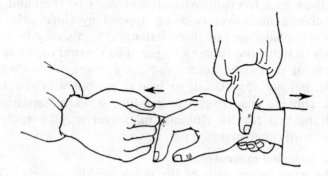

Fig. 25 Pulling maneuver

be purposely pursued, because repeated trials to obtain a crackle may cause damage to the patient's hand. The pulling maneuver may, however, be applied together with twisting and kneading maneuvers.

9. Rubbing maneuver:

A single finger or root of the palm is firmly placed on the skin at a certain point of the hand to make quick linear movement to and fro (Fig. 26) for promoting circulation of *qi* and blood, relieving stasis in collaterals, expelling cold pathogen, and toning and warming the body. The constant employment of the rubbing hand exercise may tone essence and bone marrow, prevent and treat diseases, slow the aging process, and prolong life.

Indications: The rubbing maneuver is usually applied to the fingers and palm along the direction of the bones to treat chronic diseases, cold and deficient type diseases, mental disorders, and to improve general health.

Principle of manipulation: When applying the rubbing maneuver, the wrist should be naturally extended and the hand and forearms kept in a horizontal posture. The tip of the finger applying the rubbing force may be slightly bent downward and brought to make repeated linear movement by the forearm with the elbow as a fulcrum. At different parts of the hand where the rubbing maneuver is being applied by finger, the wrist, metacarpophalangeal or interphalangeal joints may be used as an axis to move the rubbing finger. The rhythm of the rubbing movement should be quick, and the rubbing force should be gentle, but not superficial; or heavy, but not very rough. The quick rubbing maneuver can produce a warm sensation for obtaining best results. Rubbing maneuver may be applied together with other maneuvers.

10. Grinding maneuver:

The palm or the pads of the index, middle and ring fingers is placed on an area of the hand with certain acupoints for doing clockwise or counterclockwise circular movements by swinging the wrist and forearm (Fig. 27) back and forth to produce a relaxing effect after heavy manipulation. As with the rubbing maneuver, it can warm meridians, remove stagnation in collaterals, and promote circulation of *qi* and blood.

Indications: The grinding maneuver is usually applied over a wide area on the hand to treat senile, chronic cold and deficient diseases.

Principle of manipulation: The grinding movement should begin at the center of a region and gradually expanded over a

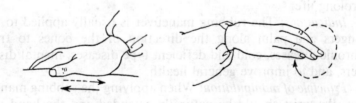

Fig. 26 Rubbing maneuver   Fig. 27 Grinding maneuver

larger and larger area, and then gradually be reduced in range and returned to the original center to produce a warm sensation over the whole area. The grinding movement should be gentle, the rhythm even, and the speed quick. The grinding force may be gradually increased, but an even and quick speed should be maintained. Otherwise, the therapeutic effect may be reduced.

II. Hand Therapy Acupuncture

Acupuncture for hand therapy includes acupuncture at regular and extra acupoints of the hand, acupuncture at reflective points of the hand, acupuncture at reflective areas of the hand, and acupuncture at special acupoints beside the second metacarpal bone. The regular and extra acupoints of the hand for hand therapy have been mentioned in Chapter 2.

1. Acupuncture at reflective points:

Acupuncture at reflective points of the hand is a type of hand therapy used to prevent and treat various diseases. According to traditional Chinese medicine, the human body is composed of Zangfu organs, meridians, five sense organs with nine orifices, four limbs, and hundreds of bones. The hands are closely related to Zangfu organs and meridians.

1) Common reflective points for acupuncture on the hand and their indications (Figs. 28 and 29):

(1) Waist point:

Location: Five cm distal to dorsal crease of wrist, on the radial side of tendon of the second digital extensor muscle and on the ulnar side of tendon of the fourth digital extensor muscle.

Indications: Lumbago and muscular sprain of waist.

(2) Hypertensive point:

Location: At the midpoint of dorsal crease of wrist.

Indication: To reduce blood pressure.

(3) Spine point:

Location: On the ulnar side of metacarpophalangeal joint of little finger and on the dorsopalmar boundary of hand.

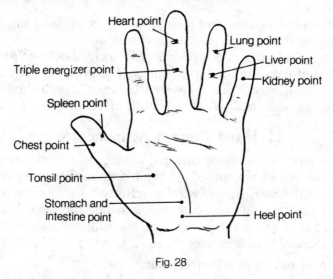

Fig. 28

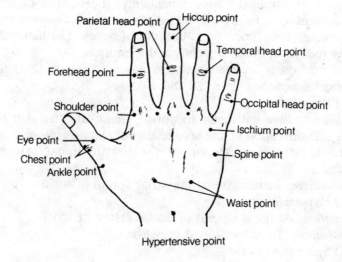

Fig. 29

Indications: Lumbago, muscular sprain of waist, and tinnitus.

(4) Ischium point:

Location: Between the fourth and fifth metacarpophalangeal joints and near the former joint.

Indications: Neuralgia, sciatica, and hip joint pain.

(5) Throat point:

Location: Between the third and fourth metacarpophalangeal joints and near the former joint.

Indications: Sore throat, toothache, and trigeminal neuralgia.

(6) Neck point:

Location: Between the second and third metacarpophalangeal joints and near the former joint.

Indications: Stiff neck and pain in neck and nape.

(7) Shoulder point:

Location: On the radial side of the second metacarpophalangeal joint and on the dorsopalmar boundary of hand.

Indications: Shoulder pain.

(8) Eye point:

Location: On the ulnar side of interphalangeal joint of thumb and on the dorsopalmar boundary of hand.

Indications: Eye diseases.

(9) Forehead point:

Location: On the radial side of proximal interphalangeal joint of index finger and on the dorsopalmar boundary of hand.

Indications: Frontal headache, diseases of stomach and intestines, and knee and ankle joint pain.

(10) Parietal head point:

Location: On the radial side of proximal interphalangeal joint of middle finger and on the dorsopalmar boundary of hand.

Indications: Parietal headache.

(11) Temporal head point:

Location: On the ulnar side of proximal interphalangeal joint of ring finger and on the dorsopalmar boundary of hand.

Indications: Migraine and chest and flank pain caused by

diseases of the liver and gallbladder.

(12) Occipital head point:

Location: On the ulnar side of proximal interphalangeal joint of little finger and on the dorsopalmar boundary of hand.

Indications: Occipital headache and tonsillitis.

(13) Hiccup point:

Location: At the midpoint of dorsal crease of distal interphalangeal of middle finger.

Indications: Hiccups.

(14) Heel point:

Location: At the midpoint of a connecting line between stomach and intestine point and Daling (PC 7) acupoint.

Indications: Heel pain.

(15) Tonsil point:

Location: On the palm and at the midpoint of ulnar border of the first metacarpal bone.

Indications: Tonsillitis and laryngitis.

(16) Stomach and intestine point:

Location: At the midpoint of a connecting line between Laogong (PC 8) and Daling (PC 7) acupoints.

Indications: Various diseases of the stomach and intestines.

(17) Ankle point:

Location: On the radial side of metacarpophalangeal joint of thumb and on the dorsopalmar boundary of hand.

Indication: Ankle joint pain.

(18) Kidney (bed-wetting) point:

Location: On the palmar surface and at the midpoint of distal interphalangeal crease of little finger.

Indications: Bed-wetting at night and frequent urination.

(19) Spleen point:

Location: On the palmar surface and at the midpoint of interphalangeal crease of thumb.

Indications: Digestive system diseases.

(20) Triple energizer point:

Location: On the palmar surface and at the midpoint of

proximal interphalangeal crease of middle finger.

Indications: Chest and abdomen diseases.

(21) Heart point:

Location: On the palmar surface and at the midpoint of distal interphalangeal crease of middle finger.

Indications: Cardiovascular diseases.

(22) Liver point:

Location: On the palmar surface and at the midpoint of proximal interphalangeal crease of ring finger.

Indications: Liver and gallbladder diseases.

(23) Lung point:

Location: On the palmar surface and at the midpoint of distal interphalangeal crease of ring finger.

Indications: Respiratory system diseases.

(24) Chest point:

Location: On the radial side of interphalangeal joint of thumb and on the dorsopalmar boundary.

Indications: Chest pain, vomiting, and diarrhea.

(25) Cough and asthma point:

Location: On the palmar surface and on the ulnar side of proximal interphalangeal joint of index finger.

Indications: Bronchitis and bronchial asthma.

(26) Toothache point: Same as throat point.

2) Acupuncture methods at reflective points:

(1) Needles 3 cm in length are used to do acupuncture.

(2) After sterilization of local skin, the needles are inserted vertically or obliquely for 1-1.6 cm in depth toward the opposite surface of hand; and after application of medium stimulation, the needles are retained for 3-5 minutes.

(3) In patients with acute muscular sprain, they are asked to move their injured part, for example the waist when the needles are twisted together with local massage. After the pain has stopped, the needling stimulation is continued for 1-3 minutes.

(4) Electrical acupuncture may be used to apply a continuous stimulation.

3) Principles of point selection:

(1) The contralateral points are usually selected in this acupuncture therapy, namely, the points on the left hand are used to treat diseases on the right side of the body, and vice versa; and the points on both hands may also be used at the same time.

(2) The points may be selected according to differential diagnosis of disease patterns in traditional Chinese medicine. For example, the liver point may be used to treat diseases of the eye, because "the eyes are the external orifice of the liver"; and the lung point may be used to treat skin diseases, because "the skin and hair are controlled by the lungs."

(3) The points may be selected according to the location of the disease. For example, the occipital point and throat point may be used to treat sore throat; the waist point may be used to treat lumbago; the eye point is used to treat eye diseases; and the shoulder point is used to treat shoulder pain.

4) Indications:

(1) This type of acupuncture can produce good analgesic effects in treating many diseases involving pain, such as pain caused by acute muscular sprain, headache, stomachache, and dysmenorrhea.

(2) It is also useful in treating oligogalactia and spasms of the eye muscles.

(3) It can be used to treat diseases curable by regular acupuncture, including cough, asthma, palpitation of heart, dizziness, diarrhea and abdominal pain.

5) Cautions:

(1) This acupuncture therapy may often produce very strong stimulation. Therefore, fainting possibly caused by this acupuncture should be avoid.

(2) The needle should not be inserted too deep, because it may injure the periosteum.

(3) The needles and local skin must be carefully sterilized to prevent infection.

6) Fainting caused by this treatment:

(1) *Causes*: This acupuncture may cause fainting if the stimulation is too strong, the patient is too tired, nervous or weak, or if acupuncture is applied while the patient is standing.

(2) *Symptoms*: The patient may suddenly develop heart palpitations, dizziness, nausea, vomiting, sweating, or even loss of consciousness.

(3) *Treatment*: The needles should be immediately removed and the patient put in a Trendelenburg's posture. A few minutes after drinking some warm water or sugar solution, the patients may recover. In severe cases, emergency drugs may be administered and acupuncture at Renzhong (GV 26) and Neiguan (PC 6) acupoints may be applied.

2. Hand therapy by acupuncture at reflective areas

This is an acupuncture therapy at the reflective areas on the hand at the miniatures of various meridians and Zangfu organs to treat general diseases of the body. It is simple, easy to learn, and effective.

1) Dividing lines for acupuncture at reflective areas:

(1) Dividing lines of *yin* and *yang*: These are the dividing boundaries of the dorsum and palm of the hand. The palmar side is *yin* and the dorsal side is *yang*.

(2) Five palmar dividing lines (Fig. 30):

First palmar line: On the palmar side, from the tip of thumb along the midline of phalangeal bones and metacarpal bone to the palmar crease of wrist at the junction one-sixth from the radial end and five-sixths from the ulnar end of the crease.

Second palmar line: On the palmar side, from the tip of index finger along the midline of phalangeal bones and metacarpal bone to the palmar crease of wrist at the junction one-third from radial end and two-thirds from the ulnar end of the crease.

Third palmar line: On the palmar side, from the tip of middle finger along the midline of phalangeal bones and metacarpal bone to the midpoint of the palmar crease of the wrist.

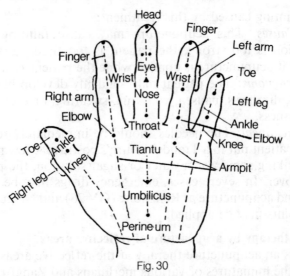

Fig. 30

Fourth palmar line: On the palmar side, from the tip of ring finger along the midline of phalangeal bones and metacarpal bone to the palmar crease of wrist at the junction two-thirds from the radial end and one-third from the ulnar end of the crease.

Fifth palmar line: On the palmar side, from the tip of little finger along the midline of phalangeal bones and metacarpal bone to the palmar crease of wrist at the junction five-sixths from the radial end and one-sixth from the ulnar end of the crease.

(3) Five dorsal dividing lines (Fig. 31):

The five dorsal dividing lines are on the dorsal side of the hand and correspond to the five palmar dividing lines on the palmar side of the hand.

2) Location of reflective areas:

(1) Dorsal reflective areas (Fig. 31):

On dorsum of left hand: The area on the ulnar side of the third dorsal line represents the dorsal side of the left half of trunk; and the area on the radial side of the third dorsal line

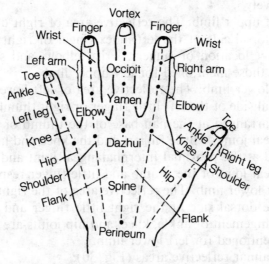

Fig. 31

represents the dorsal side of the right half of trunk.

On dorsum of right hand: The area on the ulnar side of the third dorsal line represents the dorsal side of the right half of trunk; and the area on the radial side of the third dorsal line represents the dorsal side of the left half of trunk.

Head and neck: The reflective area of head and neck is on the dorsal side of middle finger. The parietal head, occipital head, and nape are arranged symmetrically from the tip of middle finger along the third dorsal dividing line.

Trunk: The reflective area of trunk is on the dorsal side of the third metacarpal bone. The back, waist, and hip regions are arranged symmetrically from metacarpophalangeal joint to wrist joint.

Left upper limb: The reflective area of left upper limb is on the dorsal side of left ring finger or right index finger. The fingers, wrist, elbow, and shoulder are arranged at the tip of the index or ring finger, distal interphalangeal joint, proximal inter-phalangeal joint, and wrist joint of the index and ring finger respectively.

Right upper limb: The reflective area of right upper limb is on the dorsal side of the left index finger or right ring finger. The exact location of fingers, wrist, elbow, and shoulder are same as those mentioned for left upper limb.

Left lower limb: The reflective area of left lower limb is on the dorsal side of the left little finger or right thumb. The ankle joint is arranged at the nail base of the thumb or distal interphalangeal joint of little finger; and the knee and hip joints are arranged at the proximal interphalangeal joint and metacarpophalangeal joint of the thumb and little finger respectively.

Right lower limb: The reflective area of the right lower limb is on the dorsal side of the right little finger and left thumb. The arrangement of ankle, knee, and hip joints are the same as those mentioned for left lower limb.

(2) Palmar reflective areas (Fig. 30):

The reflective areas of the trunk and limbs on the palmar side of hand completely correspond to those mentioned in the dorsal reflective areas.

(3) Radial reverse dorsal reflective areas (Fig. 32):

They also represent the entire body in miniature arranged along the first and second dorsal dividing lines.

On the left hand, the ulnar side of first and second dorsal dividing lines represents the dorsal side of the left half of trunk; and the radial side of first and second dorsal dividing lines represents the dorsal side of the right half of trunk.

On the right hand, the ulnar side of first and second dorsal dividing lines represents the dorsal side of the right half of body; and the radial side of first and second dorsal dividing lines represents the dorsal side of the left half of body.

Head: The reflective area of the head is on the radial styloid process of hand.

Neck: The reflective area of the neck is over the scaphoid bone and trapezium bone.

Trunk: The reflective area of the back is on the first meta-

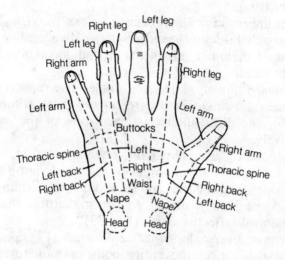

Fig. 32

carpal bone, and the spine is on the first dorsal dividing line; the lumbar and hip region is on the second metacarpal bone along the second dorsal dividing line.

Left upper limb: The reflective area of the left upper limb is on the ulnar side of the first dorsal dividing line of left hand or on the radial side of the first dorsal dividing line of the right hand.

Right upper limb: The reflective area of the right upper limb is on the radial side of the first dorsal dividing line of the left hand, or on the ulnar side of the first dorsal dividing line of the right hand.

Left and right shoulder, elbow, and wrist: The reflective areas of shoulder, elbow, and wrist joints are on the metacarpo-phalangeal and interphalangeal joints, and beside the nail bed of thumb respectively.

Left lower limb: The reflective area of the left lower limb is on the ulnar side of the second dorsal dividing line of the left hand, or on the radial side of the second dorsal dividing line of the right hand.

Right lower limb: The reflective area of the right lower limb is on the radial side of the second dorsal dividing line of the left hand, or on the ulnar side of the second dorsal dividing line of the right hand.

Left and right hip, knee, and ankle: The reflective areas of hip, knee, and ankle joints are on the metacarpophalangeal, proximal, and distal interphalangeal joint of the index finger respectively.

(4) Radial reverse palmar reflective areas:

They are the reflective areas of the trunk and limbs on the palmar side along the first and second palmar dividing lines and arranged completely similar to the miniatures of the radial reverse dorsal reflective areas (Fig. 33).

(5) Ulnar reverse dorsal reflective areas (Fig. 32):

They also reflect the entire body in miniature, arranged along the fourth and fifth dorsal dividing lines.

On the left hand, the ulnar side of the fourth and fifth dorsal

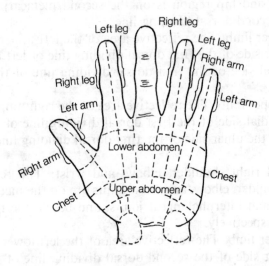

Fig. 33

dividing lines represents the dorsal side of left half of trunk; and the radial side of the fourth and fifth dorsal dividing lines represents the dorsal side of right half of trunk.

On the right hand, the ulnar side of the fourth and fifth dorsal dividing lines represents the dorsal side of right half of trunk; and the radial side of the fourth and fifth dorsal dividing lines represents the dorsal side of left half of trunk.

Head: The reflective area of the head is on the ulnar styloid process of the hand.

Neck: The reflective area of the neck is on the hamate bone.

Trunk: The reflective area of trunk is on the fifth metacarpal bone; and the reflective area of lumbar and hip region is on the fourth metacarpal bone.

Upper limb: The reflective area of both upper limbs is beside the fifth dorsal dividing line; and the reflective areas of shoulder, elbow, and wrist are on the metacarpophalangeal, proximal and distal interphalangeal joint respectively.

Lower limb: The reflective area of both lower limbs is beside the fourth dorsal dividing line; and the reflective areas of hip, knee, and ankle joints are on the metacarpophalangeal, proximal, and interphalangeal joint respectively.

(6) Ulnar reverse palmar reflective areas:

They are the reflective areas of trunk and limbs on the palmar side and the ulnar half of the hand, and arranged completely similar to the miniature of the ulnar reverse dorsal reflective areas (Fig. 33).

3) Functions and indications of reflective areas:

(1) Dorsal reflective areas, radial reverse dorsal reflective areas, and ulnar reverse dorsal reflective areas: They can adjust and regulate locomotive functions and treat diseases of the nervous, circulatory, and locomotive systems as well as diseases on the dorsal side of the body.

(2) Palmar reflective areas, radial reverse palmar reflective areas, and ulnar reverse palmar reflective areas: They can adjust and regulate sensory functions and treat pain, numbness,

and disturbances of hot and cold skin sensations, as well as diseases of the internal organs and those on the ventral side of the body.

4) Principles for selecting reflective areas:

(1) According to the location of disease: The reflective area of the waist in radial reverse dorsal reflective areas is selected for treating lumbago.

(2) According to the meridian theory: The reflective area of the left shoulder in radial reverse dorsal reflective areas is selected for treating diseases of the right shoulder.

5) Combined selection of reflective areas:

(1) The dorsal reflective areas, radial reverse dorsal reflective areas, and ulnar reverse dorsal reflective areas may be used in combinations.

(2) The palmar reflective areas, radial reverse palmar reflective areas, and ulnar reverse palmar reflective areas may be used in combinations.

(3) The reflective areas on dorsal and palmar side of the hand may also be used in combinations.

6) Method of manipulation: The needles, 3 cm in length, are quickly and vertically punctured into the skin, either superficially or deeply to reach the periosteum. They are removed right after stimulation by twisting, thrusting, and lifting the needles. The duration of treatment is determined by the nature of the disease.

7) Precautions:

(1) Needles and skin must be carefully sterilized.

(2) Because this treatment may produce very strong stimulation, fainting should be carefully guarded against (refer to the cautions in Acupuncture at Reflective Points for Hand Therapy).

3. Hand therapy by acupuncture at special acupoints beside the second metacarpal bone

This is a hand therapy employing acupuncture, massage or pressure to treat general diseases of the body.

1) Theoretical basis:

(1) The hand Yangming large intestine meridian passes through the region beside the second metacarpal bone and it is externally and internally related to the hand Taiyin lung meridian, and also closely related to the foot Yangming stomach meridian. The hand Taiyin lung meridian is the beginning as well as the end of the meridional cycle, composed of 12 meridians. Therefore, treatment applied beside the second metacarpal bone can cure general diseases of the body.

(2) According to the theory of biological homography, the region beside the second metacarpal bone is a miniature of the human body.

2) Commonly used acupoints and their indications:

With the hand clenched to make a hollow fist, the 12 special acupoints of the head, neck, upper limb, lung and heart, liver, stomach, duodenum, kidney, waist, lower abdomen, leg, and foot are arranged in sequence beside the second metacarpal bone.

(1) Head acupoint:

Location: At the junction of radial end of the crease passing through the center of palm with the radial border of the second metacarpal bone.

Indications: Diseases of head, eye, ear, nose, mouth and teeth.

(2) Neck acupoint:

Location: Between the head acupoint and upper limb acupoint.

Indications: Diseases of neck and nape, thyroid gland, pharynx, upper segment of trachea, and esophagus.

(3) Upper limb acupoint:

Location: Between neck acupoint and lung and heart acupoint.

Indications: Diseases of shoulder, upper limb, elbow, wrist, hand, and middle segment of esophagus.

(4) Lung and heart acupoint:

Location: At the midpoint between the head acupoint and the stomach acupoint.

Indications: Diseases of lung, heart, chest, breast, lower segment of trachea and bronchus, lower segment of esophagus, and back.

(5) Liver acupoint:

Location: At the midpoint between the lung and heart acupoint and the stomach acupoint.

Indications: Diseases of the liver and gallbladder.

(6) Stomach acupoint:

Location: At the midpoint between the head acupoint and the foot acupoint.

Indications: Diseases of stomach, spleen and pancreas.

(7) Duodenum acupoint:

Location: Between the stomach acupoint and the kidney acupoint.

Indications: Diseases of duodenum and right flexure of colon.

(8) Kidney acupoint:

Location: Between duodenum acupoint and waist acupoint.

Indications: Diseases of kidney and small and large intestines.

(9) Waist acupoint:

Location: At the midpoint between the stomach acupoint and the foot acupoint.

Indications: Diseases of waist, periumbilical region, and large and small intestines.

(10) Lower abdomen acupoint:

Location: Between waist acupoint and leg acupoint.

Indications: Diseases of lower abdomen, sacrum, uterus, urinary bladder, rectum, appendix, ovary, vagina, testis, urethra, and anus.

(11) Leg acupoint:

Location: Between lower abdomen acupoint and foot acupoint.

Indications: Diseases of the leg and knee.

(12) Foot acupoint:

Location: At the junction of the first and second metacarpal bones, and near the former.

Indications: Diseases of the foot and ankle.

3) Exact localization of acupoint: The tip of thumb or a probe is used to press from the head acupoint along the line of acupoints beside the second metacarpal bone, 1-3 times at each spot. Once an apparent sensation of soreness, numbness, heaviness or pain is detected, this tender spot is the exact location of an acupoint.

4) Principles for selection of acupoint:

(1) According to the location of disease: The head acupoint is selected for headache; and the lung and heart acupoint for chest pain.

(2) According to the theory of traditional Chinese medicine, the heart can control mental activity and blood vessels, the condition of the heart is reflected on the face, and its indicator is the tongue. Therefore, the heart acupoint is used to treat diseases of the mind, blood vessels, and the tongue. The liver can store blood and control ligaments, the condition of the liver is reflected on the nails, and its orifice is the eye. Therefore, the liver point is used to treat diseases of the blood, ligaments, nails, and eye. The spleen is a foundation for the development and growth of the body after birth and it can control the muscles. The condition of the spleen is shown on the lips. Therefore, the spleen (stomach) acupoint can be used to treat diseases of the digestive system, muscles, and lips. The lung can control the skin and hair and its orifice is the nose. Therefore, the lung acupoint can be used to treat diseases of the skin, hair, and nose. The orifice of the kidney is the ear. Therefore, the kidney acupoint can be used to treat diseases of the ear.

(3) Both ipsilateral or bilateral acupoints can be selected to treat disease on one side of the body.

5) Method of manipulation:

(1) A 3-cm-long needle is inserted at the tender spot along the radial border of the second metacarpal bone toward the center of the palm for 1.6-2.6 cm.

(2) During the 30 minutes the needle is kept in place, the stimulation may be repeated 2-3 times to maintain the needling sensation. Acupuncture is applied once a day for seven days as a therapeutic course.

(3) Acupuncture may produce a good therapeutic effect if a local hot sensation or sweating appears 10 minutes after the needling stimulation.

(4) Instead of acupuncture, the finger or a probe may be used to press or to knead the tender spot clockwise or counterclockwise with a frequency of 100 per minute for 3-5 minutes to produce a sore, numb, heavy and distending sensation. The pressure should not be very heavy and the duration of the massage should not be very long to avoid damaging the skin.

(5) Pressure applied with beans: According to the stage of the disease, the proper acupoints are selected for application of mung beans or vaccaria seeds, fixed by adhesive plaster. The beans or seeds are pressed and kneaded to produce stimulation at the acupoints, and the acupoints on both hands may be used alternately for two weeks as a therapeutic course. The duration of stimulation and therapy is determined by the nature of the disease. This is a simple, painless treatment which can produce good results if the location of the acupoint is correct.

6) *Indications*: This therapy has wide indications, including neurasthenia, spasms of the facial muscles, diseases of the ear, eye, nose and pharynx, paraplegia, pain in limbs, common cold, trigeminal neuralgia, facial palsy, stiff neck, vertigo, frozen shoulder, diseases of the oral cavity, bronchitis, hypertension, angina pectoris, heart arrhythmia, liver and gallbladder disease, stomach spasms, gastric ulcer, acute and chronic enteritis, diarrhea, dysentery, hiccups, diabetes mellitus, acute waist sprain, soft tissue injury, rheumatism, neuralgia sciatica, renal diseases, incontinence of urine, emission, irregular menstruation, and

vaginitis.

7) Precautions:

(1) This is a therapy with strong stimulation. Therefore, fainting should be carefully avoided (refer to the precautions in Hand Therapy by Acupuncture at Regular and Extra Acupoints).

(2) The acupoints should be correctly localized at the most painful tender spots.

(3) Generally, 1-3 acupoints are enough for one treatment.

III. Hand Therapy Using Hand Bath

Hand bath is a steaming and washing therapy. The hot steam from an herbal decoction is used to heat the hands which are then soaked in the warm decoction after it gradually cools down. Diseases can be cured by the hot stimulation applied to the meridians and acupoints of the hand and by the gradual absorption of herbs through the skin.

1. Origin and classification of steaming and washing therapy:
Steaming and washing therapy originated in ancient times. Among 52 ancient herbal therapy recipes unearthed from the Han Dynasty Mawangdui Tomb, eight were used for steaming and washing therapy. This indicates that steaming and washing therapy has been used by Chinese people to treat diseases for at least 2,000 years. This therapy is also mentioned in classical medical books of the Han (206 B. C.-220) and Jin (265-420) dynasties. During the Tang Dynasty (618-907), this method was used to treat carbuncles, cellulitis, skin rashes, dermatitis, frostbite, hand and foot diseases, and gynecological and eye disorders. In the Kin (1115-1234) and Yuan (1271-1368) dynasties this method was classified as an essential medical therapy. In the Qing Dynasty (1644-1911)), Wu Shangxian, a famous physician of traditional Chinese medicine, divided this therapy into smoking, steaming, shower, sitz bath, and hot ironing. It is a folk treatment used by common people to treat acute sprains, bone injuries, and contusions with a good therapeutic results.

Steaming and washing therapy can be classified as general and local. Local treatment includes steaming and washing therapy for the hand, foot, and eye, and sitz baths. Hand bath is steaming and washing therapy for the hand.

2. Function and characteristics of hand bath:

As demonstrated by the experiments of modern medicine, steaming and washing therapy with hot and moist air can promote the absorption of herbs through the skin, dilate the skin's small blood vessels, promote the circulation of blood and lymph, enhance the phagocytic functions of the reticuloendothelial system, increase the permeability of cellular membranes, and promote metabolism by stimulating the sensitive sensory nerves scattered along the skin. The effective components of herbs used in steaming and washing therapy can directly kill the pathogenic germs on the skin. According to the theory of traditional medicine, the meridians of the hand are closely related to the organs and meridians of the entire body. Therefore, this therapy can clear stagnation in meridians, adjust bodily deficiency and excess, and promote circulation of qi and blood.

The hand bath is simple, cheap, and easy to learn and practice, with numerous indications and good therapeutic effects, and without any harmful side effects. It is most useful for patients proscribed from taking drugs.

3. Methods of manipulation:

1) The proper recipe is selected according to the diseases and the basin, towel and sheets are prepared in use.

2) The hot decoction of herbs is poured into the basin and the hands and arms are put over the basin. Cover the arms and basin with a sheet to reserve the hot air from quickly escaping away. Some boiled water may be added to the basin to maintain the temperature. After the decoction is cooled down to an adequate temperature, the hands may be soaked and washed in the decoction.

3) After steaming and bathing, the hands should be dried

with a towel and protected from attack of wind and coldness.

4) The steaming and washing therapy may last for 20-30 minutes, twice a day.

4. Precautions:

1) The water used to boil the herbs should be adequate to prepare a decoction of the proper concentration. Aromatic and volatile herbs should be boiled for only 10-15 minutes; and roots, stems and herbs in large clumps should be boiled for 30 minutes.

2) The temperature of the decoction for bathing and soaking the hands should be monitored to avoid burning the skin.

3) These decoctions are not for oral administration.

IV. Hand Therapy Using Hand *Qigong*

Hand *qigong* is employed as physical exercises of the hand or the entire body induced by the hand, and is usually accompanied by breathing and mental exercises for treating diseases.

1. Origin and classification of hand *qigong*

Hand *qigong* is a branch of medical *qigong* for treatment of diseases and has a long developing history. There were an introduction and case reports mentioned in the medical literature of the Sui (581-618), Tang, Ming (1368-1644), and Qing dynasties.

Hand *qigong* can be divided into two types: The pure physical exercise of the hand for treating diseases of the internal organs, and exercises of the entire body induced by the hand with breathing and mental exercises to adjust meridians, *qi*, and blood throughout the body.

2. Function and characteristics of hand *qigong*

The hand is closely connected to tissues and organs of the entire body through meridians, and there are many sensitive and effective acupoints, such as Hegu (LI 4), Laogong (PC 8) and Shaoshang (LU 11) on the hand. Therefore, the physical exercises of the hand and physical exercises of the body induced by the hand with breathing and mental exercises can adjust *qi*, breath and mental activity, promote circulation of *qi* and blood through meridians, adjust deficiency and excess in internal organs, and balance *yin* and *yang* throughout the body.

This exercise is simple, practical, easy to learn, and can be practiced by people of all ages at any time and place. It is effective for treating many diseases, especially chronic diseases, without harmful side effects.

3. Precautions:

Before doing *qigong* exercises the practitioner should get rid of mental distractions, maintain a calm mental state, assume a proper posture, and develop a slow and even breath. Then, various types of special hand exercises or physical exercises of the entire body may begin.

Practical methods of *qigong* exercises will be discussed in the treatment of different diseases included in the following chapter.

V. Hand Therapy Using Miscellaneous Methods

Besides massage, acupuncture, hand bath, and hand *qigong*, there are some other therapies applied to or near the hand including holding herbs, pressing and kneading maneuvers applied along the second metacarpal bone, swinging arms, and playing bracelet or ball with the hand.

1. Holding herb therapy

As an external treatment herbs, properly selected according to the nature of the disease, are held in the hand as a treatment for various ailments.

This is an ancient therapy. Herbs that induce sweating and promote digestion are best absorbed through the skin of a hot and moist palm to stimulate the meridians and acupoints of the hand.

Herbs for particular diseases come in a variety of shapes and patterns such as pills or powders, easy to hold in the hand.

Fresh raw herbs are also produced for therapeutic use. Before holding the herbs, the hands should be soaked in hot water for a while. The herbs are then held in the hand until a slight sweating is induced. The herbs should be wrapped in gauze and secured to the palm by bandage for babies and young children.

This method is used to treat common colds, headache, facial palsy, and indigestion in children.

Corrosive or allergenic herbs should not be used, and it is contraindicated for patients with ulcers or wounds of the palm.

2. Pressing and kneading therapy beside the second metacarpal bone

The pressing and kneading maneuvers are applied at the points on the radial side of the second metacarpal bone for treating various diseases.

The location, indications, and principles for selecting points have been discussed in Acupuncture for Hand Therapy.

The pressing and kneading maneuvers are chiefly applied in an area around Hegu (LI 4) acupoint. The Hegu acupoint is an important point used to control pain all over the body and is especially effective for stopping pain of the head and face and in the chest, abdomen, and upper and lower limbs.

The patient is asked to relax the hand muscles and make a hollow fist with the radial side facing upward. The physician holds the patient's fist by one hand and applies pressure with some kneading movement at a frequency of 150 per minute at Hegu acupoint with the thumb of the other hand to produce a sore, distending, heavy, and numb sensation for three minutes.

The point should be correctly located; the pressure should be vertically applied to a deep layer, and should be gentle to avoid damaging the skin.

3. Swinging arm exercise

This exercise was developed and taught by Mr. Tian Ruifang in Shanghai, 1961. It is a physical exercise, simple and easy to learn and practice and effective for treating certain chronic diseases.

1) Preparation: Before starting the exercise, the practitioner should be rid of all mental distractions, calm the mind, and fully relax every part of the body and remain this way for 3-5 minutes.

2) Posture:

(1) The feet are separated to a distance the width of the shoulders to maintain a natural stance, with the head and body kept erect, the knees naturally and slightly flexed, and the arms freely dangling down (Fig. 34).

(2) The neck is relaxed, the chin is held slightly backward and the vortex of the head, Baihui (GV 20) acupoint (at midpoint between bilateral tips of ear auricle), is intentionally raised upward.

(3) The pectoralis major muscles are relaxed and the shoulders are slightly drawn forward to draw in the chest and straighten the back and to produce a counteraction against the intentional upward ascent of the vortex of the head. The qi may move downward to Dantian when the chest is drawn in; and the qi may diffuse all over the abdomen when the abdomen is relaxed. After the clear qi is moved upward and the dirty qi is moved downward, a result of "deficiency in upper part and excessiveness in lower part of body" can occur.

(4) The shoulders are relaxed and sagging to draw in the chest and move the qi downward to Dantian. Otherwise, the qi may move upward, if the shoulders are shrugged.

(5) The thigh, leg, and foot are all relaxed.

(6) The muscles all over the body are relaxed with a smiling face and a generally comfortable demeanor.

(7) The tongue should be naturally flat in the mouth. The mouth and teeth should be lightly closed, because the mouth and tongue may become dry if the mouth is opened; and the practitioner cannot relax the body if the mouth is tightly closed and the teeth gnashed.

3) Method of performance:

(1) Both naturally extended arms are moved forward with

the shoulder joints as a fulcrum, the fingers are naturally and comfortably extended, the palms are slightly concave and facing forward, and the thumbs are slightly flexed and pointing downward. The hands are moved forward and upward, but not beyond the umbilicus (Fig. 35).

(2) The shoulders are relaxed and the arms swing freely backward to the initial position, but not beyond the buttocks, with the shape of the palms unchanged (Fig. 36). The forward and backward movement of the arms are continuously repeated.

(3) The arms are moved back and forth by the relaxed shoulders. The shoulders should not be shrugged and the arms always move parallel. The arms are moved forward by a force conducted from the shoulder and then freely swung backward by gravity, as a repeated movement with arms alternately kept tense and relaxed.

(4) The palms are slightly concave and the fingers are slightly flexed and separated, because the full extension of tight fingers may interfere with meridians and the free circulation of internal *qi*.

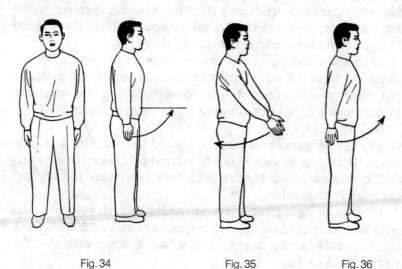

Fig. 34   Fig. 35   Fig. 36

(5) The arms should be naturally extended throughout the back and forth movement and the elbows should not be flexed to move the forearms alone.

(6) The feet are flat on the ground. With increased experience, the practitioner may keep a stance with the toes firmly holding the ground.

(7) The swinging arm exercise should be carried with the body relaxed, quiet, and natural.

4) Repetitions, speed, and silent counting:

(1) Repetitions: The arms may be moved back and forth repeatedly 2,000 times each morning and evening. Beginners may start their exercise with several hundred repetitions according to their physique, and gradually increase the number.

(2) Speed: An adequate speed is 2,000 repetitions in 40 minutes. The practitioner may choose a proper speed for themselves to produce a comfortable feeling and maintain this fixed speed day by day through the entire course of exercise. The purpose of this external exercise is to induce a correspondent internal exercise within the body, and the establishment of this internal exercise depends on a rhythmic external exercise. So the internal exercise is difficult to induce and establish if the speed of the external exercise is constantly changed.

(3) Silent counting of repetitions: In order to concentrate the mind and be rid of mental distractions, the numbers are silently but clearly and conscientiously counted when the arms are moved forward, but not counted while swinging backward.

5) Precautions:

(1) The swinging arm exercise should be practiced in a calm mode. Therefore, it should not be started before extreme mental and emotional disturbances, like fury, joy, and anxiety are completely controlled.

(2) The swinging arm exercise should be performed in good weather when outdoors and in a quiet environment with fresh air. It should not be practiced in a bad weather with thunder storms or thick fog.

(3) The swinging arm exercise should be done wearing large and loose-fitting clothes. Before beginning, the neck button should be unbuttoned, the belt loosened, and eyeglasses removed.

(4) For patients with internal organ diseases, the exercise should be practiced gently. But following improvement and increased experience, the exercise may be gradually done more and more vigorously.

(5) During the exercise, some parts of the body may become numb, distended, hot, or aching, and the practitioner may belch, experience abdominal gurgling, or break wind. These are normal responses and an indication of the *qi* accumulating phenomenon. It is not necessary to either worry about it or purposely induce or seek it. Otherwise, the normal practice of this exercise may be disturbed. In addition, after practicing for several days, a numb, hot or aching sensation may be detected in the soles of the feet. Exercise should nevertheless continue at the same place and in the same posture. Otherwise, the effect of the exercise may be reduced.

(6) Sometimes, the practitioner may make spontaneous swinging movements, without intentional control. This may be allowed to go with the natural tendency of its development. The practitioner has no reason to worry about it or to purposely continue or promptly stop it. If the practitioner felt tired, he (or she) may purposely slow down the spontaneous swinging movement so as to finally stop the movement.

(7) The exercise should be stopped if the practitioner becomes dizzy or has other bodily discomforts. It may be resumed the next day after the discomfort disappears.

(8) After practicing this exercise for a period of time, the appetite, sleep, and physical strength will all be much improved. It may also produce good therapeutic effects for treating neurasthenia, stomach diseases, frozen shoulder, arthritis, pulmonary tuberculosis, bronchitis and asthma; and many also be found to be useful in treating hypertension, liver diseases and

heart diseases, if the patient strictly follows the regulations for practicing this exercise.

4. Playing hand bracelet or hand ball therapy

These hand bracelets (Fig. 37) and hand balls are small health-maintaining instruments which can produce good effects for improving life quality and maintaining health through the exercise of the hand and stimulation applied to meridians and acupoints. These exercises can remove stagnation from meridians and promote the circulation of *qi* and blood.

The hand bracelets are rubber wheels that come in large, medium, and small sizes for people with hands in different sizes and there are many granules scattered on their surface. The elastic bracelet may be held in the palm and repeatedly and rhythmically squeezed and released. The granules produce a massage effect to stimulate many acupoints on the palm for promoting the circulation of *qi* and blood, improving movement of joints, and refreshing mental activities.

The hand balls are paired balls made of rock crystal, stone, glass or metal (stainless steel, bronze or iron) with a smooth surface, also called mother-child or male-female balls. They are manufactured in sizes suitable for all. The balls are nimbly rotated in one or both hands to press and knead the palm acupoints for relaxing muscles, promoting circulation of blood,

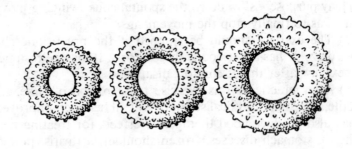

Fig. 37

improving movement of joints, refreshing mental activity, and retarding the aging process. The number of balls rotated in each hand may be gradually increased from two to as many as eight, as the user becomes more skilful. The hand ball exercise may be performed along with elegant gymnastics as a physical exercise and an enjoyment of art, beneficial for both body and mind.

Chapter 4
TREATMENT OF COMMON DISEASES

I. Medical Diseases

1. Common cold
The common cold is a disease caused by an attack of external pathogens, occurring in all four seasons but more frequently in winter and spring. The clinical symptoms include nasal obstruction, running nose, sneezing, cough, headache, chills, fever and general discomfort. This disease can be divided into mild and heavy types: The mild type is called the common cold, caused by current pathogens; the heavy type is called influenza, caused by unseasonable pathogens; and the epidemic type with similar symptoms shared by many patients and occurring in one seasonal epidemic is called epidemic influenza.

In modern medicine, upper respiratory infection and epidemic influenza are included as variants of this disease and can be treated by the following methods.

Applications of hand therapy:

1) Massage therapy:

Location: Thenar prominence, Hegu (LI 4), head reflective point, lung and heart acupoint, lung area, nose and throat area, chest area, dorsal side of the third metacarpal bone, antifebrile point and Taiyuan (LU 9).

Method of manipulation: Pinching and digit-pressing maneuvers applied at Hegu, head point and lung and heart acupoint; pressing and kneading maneuvers at lung area, nose and throat area and chest area; rubbing palm and dorsal side of the third metacarpal bone; digit-pressing at antifebrile point, Taiyuan and Shangyang (LI 1) for 30-50 times at each point and area.

2) Acupuncture therapy:

(1) At regular and extra acupoints:

Location: Quchi (LI 11), Waiguan (TE 5) and Hegu (LI 4).

Method of manipulation: The needles are vertically inserted to apply medium stimulation.

(2) At reflective point:

Location: Lung point.

Method of manipulation: The needle is vertically inserted for 1.6 cm and retained for 15 minutes after twisting, lifting, and thrusting needling stimulation.

(3) At reflective areas:

Location: Head area and neck area of dorsal reflective areas.

Method of manipulation: The area is superficially pricked with a 3.3-cm-long needle. The needle is not retained.

(4) At special acupoints beside the second metacarpal bone:

Location: Head acupoint and lung acupoint.

Method of manipulation: Strong stimulation is applied and the needles are retained for 20 minutes.

3) Hand bath:

Recipe: Mahuang (Herba Ephedrae) 10 g, Guizhi (Ramulus Cinnomomi) 10 g, Jingjie (Herba Schizonepetae) 15 g, Zisu (Leaf of Perilla) 15 g, Qianghuo (Radix Notopterygii) 15 g, Huajiao (Pericarpium Zanthoxyli) 6 g, fresh stalks of green onion 30 g, and fresh ginger 10 g.

Function: To induce sweating by pungent and warm herbs, improve ventilation of lungs, and relieve symptoms of exterior syndrome.

Method of manipulation: A hot decoction of these herbs is used to steam and then wash both hands, head and face for 20-30 minutes, twice a day, for treating common cold due to an attack of wind and cold pathogens, but not due to wind and heat pathogens.

4) Herb-holding therapy:

Herbs: Cangzhu (Rhizoma Atractylodis) 6 g, Qianghuo (Radix Notopterygii) 10 g, Mingfan (Alumen) 6 g and Jingjie (Herba Schizonepetae) 9 g.

Method of manipulation: A powder of these herbs is mixed with ginger juice to prepare pills for holding in palm to slightly induce sweating, three times a day for treating common cold due to an attack of wind and cold pathogens.

2. Cough

Coughing is an important symptom of respiratory system diseases. In traditional Chinese medicine, a cough without sputum is called *ke*; and the spitting of sputum without a cough is called *sou*. Usually coughing and spitting sputum are present at the same time.

In modern medicine, the cough is included as part of respiratory diseases such as acute and chronic bronchitis, bronchiectasis, and pneumonia and can be treated by the following methods.

Applications of hand therapy:

1) Massage therapy:

Location: Taiyuan (LU 9), Yuji (LU 10), Shaofu (HT 8), lung reflective point, cough-controlling point, Shaoshang (LU 11), Hegu (LI 4), Sifeng (EX-UE 10), nose and throat area, lung area and thenar prominence.

Method of manipulation: Digit-pressing and kneading maneuvers applied at Taiyuan (LU 9), Yuji (LU 10), Shaofu (HT 8), lung point, Shaoshang (LU 11) and Hegu (LI 4); pinching maneuver at Sifeng (EX-UE-10); and pressing and grinding maneuvers at nose and throat area, lung area and thenar prominence. Body warmth should be maintained, and the pressing and kneading maneuvers should be applied to the deep part of the hand, and the rubbing and grinding maneuvers should heat and redden the skin.

2) Acupuncture therapy:

(1) At regular and extra acupoints:

Location: Lieque (LU 7) and Chize (LU 5).

Method of manipulation: The medium needling stimulation is applied and the needles are retained for 30 minutes.

(2) At reflective points:

Location: Cough and asthma point and lung point.

Method of manipulation: The needles are inserted for 1.6 cm in depth and retained for five minutes after twisting, lifting, and thrusting stimulation.

(3) At reflective area:

Location: Lung area in palmar reflective areas.

Method of manipulation: The needle is shallowly inserted and removed after lifting and thrusting stimulation.

(4) At special acupoint beside the second metacarpal bone:

Location: Lung acupoint.

Method of manipulation: The needle is inserted for 3.3 cm and retained for 30 minutes.

3) Hand bath:

(1) For cough caused by wind cold pathogens:

Recipe: Mahuang (Herba Ephedrae) 15 g, Xingren (Semen Armeniacae Amarum) 15 g, Zisu (Leaf of Perilla) 30 g, Baibu (Radix Stemonae) 20 g, Qianhu (Radix Peucedani Cirrhosae) 15 g, and fresh ginger 10 g.

Function: To relieve symptoms of exterior syndrome, improve ventilation of lung, and control cough.

Method of manipulation: A hot decoction of these herbs is used to steam and then wash both hands for 20-30 minutes, twice a day.

(2) Cough due to internal injury:

Recipe: Xingren (Semen Armeniacae Amarum) 20 g, Baibu (Radix Stemonae) 20 g, Gouqizi (Fructus Lycii) 20 g, Dangshen (Radix Codonopsis Pilosulae) 20 g, Danggui (Chinese angelica) 30 g, Jiegeng (Radix Platycodi) 30 g and Gancao (Licorice root) 10 g.

Function: To improve body resistance, tone the body, resolve phlegm and control cough.

Method of manipulation: Same as above recipe.

3. Shortness of breath

Patients usually have shortness of breath or difficulty breathing with repeated elevation of shoulders and flaring nostrils. The patient often cannot lie flat and severe cases may include develop fainting. This is a symptom of many acute and chronic diseases.

In modern medicine, shortness of breath or difficulty breathing occurs in acute and chronic bronchitis, infection of lungs, pneumonia, pulmonary emphysema, chronic pulmonary heart disease, and cardiac failure. These can be treated by the following methods.

Applications of hand therapy:

1) Massage therapy:

Location: Shaoshang (LU 11), Taiyuan (LU 9), cough and asthma point, asthma-controlling point, lung reflective point, lung area, throat area, chest and diaphragm area, thenar prominence, and ring finger.

Method of manipulation: Pressing and kneading maneuvers applied at Taiyuan (LU 9), cough and asthma point and asthma-controlling point; pinching maneuver at lung point; and pressing and kneading maneuvers at Shaoshang (LU 11). Heavy manipulation may be applied at the tender spots and the intensity of manipulation may be reduced to medium and gentle levels when the symptoms are alleviated.

2) Acupuncture therapy:

(1) At regular and extra acupoints:

Location: Yuji (LU 10) and Taiyuan (LU 9).

Method of manipulation: The needles are inserted for 3.3 cm and retained for 20 minutes after twisting, lifting, and thrusting stimulation.

(2) At reflective points:

Location: Lung point and cough and asthma point.

Method of manipulation: The needles are inserted for 1.6 cm and retained for five minutes after twisting, lifting, and thrusting stimulation.

(3) At reflective areas:

Location: Lung area at palmar reflective areas, ulnar reverse palmar, and radial reverse palmar reflective areas.

Method of manipulation: The needles are shallowly inserted and then removed after twisting, lifting, and thrusting stimulation.

(4) At special acupoints beside the second metacarpal bone:

Location: Lung acupoint and kidney acupoint.

Method of manipulation: The needles are inserted for 3.3 cm and retained for 30 minutes.

3) Hand bath:

Recipe: Mahuang (Herba Ephedrae) 20 g, Xingren (Semen Armeniacae Amarum) 20 g, Baiguo (ginkgo seeds) 15 g, Ziyuan (Radix Asteris) 20 g, Houpo (Magnolia bark) 15 g and Gancao (licorice root) 10 g.

Function: To improve ventilation of lungs, promote downward transportation of *qi*, and control cough and asthma.

Method of manipulation: A hot decoction of these herbs is used to steam and wash both hands for 30 minutes, twice a day.

4) Hand *qigong*:

(1) Physical and breathing exercise for asthma:

The patient sits in an erect position with both legs or one leg crossed, or in a lying posture on either side. If in a sitting posture, the hands hold each other and one thumb is pressed at Laogong (PC 8) acupoint of the other hand; in a lying posture, the head and neck are kept in a neutral posture at an adequate height with the head bent slightly forward; and the spine is bent slightly forward with the shoulders rounded and the back stretched. If lying on the right side, the right upper limb is naturally flexed with the fingers flexed slightly and the palm is placed near the face on the pillow and facing upward; the left upper limb is naturally extended and placed on the hip, and the palm over the thigh with the fingers separated; the right lower limb is naturally extended and the left knee joint is flexed to 120 degrees. If lying on the left side, the position of all four limbs is reversed. Both eyes are closed and breathing is natural; attention is concentrated on the navel as if looking at a red light radiating from light bulb. The brightness of the light is gradually increased and the irradiating scope of the light is gradually expanded to the trunk, limbs, and fingers. This mental exercise may be repeated several times (Fig. 38).

(2) Kongjin exercise (exercise with potential strength): The hand is prone with palm facing downward and fingers extended and relaxed. The thumb and middle fingers are simultaneously flexed (Fig. 39) nine times. After each movement, the hand resumes a ladder pattern. The little finger is flexed twice and the hand again resumes a ladder pattern. The exercise is ended after a pole-standing exercise in riding posture for five minutes.

4. Asthma

Asthma is a disease characterized by paroxysmal attacks of gasping, difficulty breathing, and a whistling noise in the throat. Victims of these attacks are often unable to lie flat. The disease is caused by an accumulation of phlegm, constriction of the respiratory tract, and interference with pulmonary ventilation

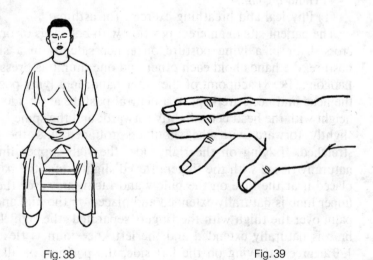

Fig. 38   Fig. 39

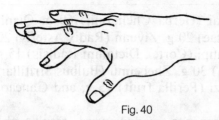

Fig. 40

producing gasps and a whistling sound.

Bronchial asthma, asthmatic bronchitis, and asthmatic attacks due to other diseases such as pulmonary emphysema, bronchiectasis, chronic bronchitis, rheumatic heart disease, and eosinophilia in modern medicine can be treated by the following methods.

Applications of hand therapy:

1) Acupuncture therapy:

(1) At regular and extra acupoints:

Location: Neiguan (PC 6), Chize (LU 5) and Taiyuan (LU 9) acupoints.

Method of manipulation: The needles are vertically inserted for 3.3 cm and retained for 20 minutes after medium needling stimulation.

(2) At reflective points:

Location: Cough and asthma point and lung point.

Method of manipulation: The needles are inserted for 1.6 cm and retained for five minutes after twisting, lifting, and thrusting needling stimulation.

(3) At reflective areas:

Location: Lung area of palmar reflective and radial reverse palmar reflective areas.

Method of manipulation: The needles are shallowly inserted and removed after twisting, lifting, and thrusting stimulation.

(4) At special acupoints beside the second metacarpal bone:

Location: Lung acupoint and stomach acupoint.

Method of manipulation: The needles are inserted for 3.3 cm and retained for 30 minutes.

2) Hand bath:

Recipe: Baiqucai (Herba Chelidonii) 60 g, Qianhu (Radix Peucedani Cirrhosae) 20 g, Ziyuan (Radix Asteris) 20 g, earthworm 15 g, Baixianpi (Cortex Dictamni Radicis) 15 g, Kushen (Shrubby Sophora) 30 g, Zhebeimu (Bulbus Stritillariae Thunbergii) 15 g, Zisuzi (Perilla fruit) 15 g, and Gancao (Licorice root) 15 g.

Function: To transport *qi* downward, resolve phlegm, and control cough and asthma.

Method of manipulation: The herbs are boiled in water for 40-60 minutes and the hot decoction in a basin is used to steam and then wash both hands for 20-30 minutes, two to three times a day.

3) Hand *qigong*: Kongjin exercise.

The hand is prone with palm facing downward and fingers extended and relaxed. The thumb and ring finger are repeatedly flexed at same time (Fig. 40) for nine repetitions, and after each movement the hand resumes the original ladder pattern; the middle finger is flexed for three times and the hand again resumes its ladder pattern. The exercise is ended after a pole-standing exercise in the riding posture for five minutes.

5. Heart palpitations

This is a disease characterized by attacks of fright and anxiety with rapid heart beat and sometimes loss of self-control, usually caused by emotional disturbance or overfatigue and often accompanied by insomnia, poor memory, vertigo, and tinnitus.

Cardiac arrhythmia due to various causes, including tachycardia, bradycardia, presystole, auricular fibrillation and flutter, auriculoventricular block, sick sinus syndrome, pre-excitation syndrome, heart failure, myocarditis, pericarditis, and neurasthenia in modern medicine may be treated by the following methods.

Applications of hand therapy:

1) Massage therapy:

Location: Entire palm, either side of little finger, heart area, kidney area, cardiac palpitation point, Shenmen (HT 7), Shaofu (HT 8), Daling (PC 7) and Shaochong (HT 9).

Method of manipulation: Forcibly rubbing entire palm, rubbing and kneading central part of palm, and rubbing either side of little finger to produce a hot sensation; pressing central part of palm, heart area and kidney area; digit-pressing and kneading maneuvers applied at Shenmen (HT 7), Shaofu (HT 8), Daling (PC 7) and Shaochong (HT 9); and pinching and kneading at cardiac palpitation point. The manipulation should be gently applied and body warmth should be maintained.

2) Acupuncture therapy:

(1) At regular and extra acupoints:

Location: Neiguan (PC 6) and Shenmen (HT 7) acupoints.

Method of manipulation: The needles are inserted for 1.6 cm and retained for 30 minutes.

(2) At reflective point:

Location: Heart point.

Method of manipulation: The needle is inserted for 1.6 cm and retained for five minutes.

(3) At reflective area:

Location: Heart area of palmar reflective areas.

Method of manipulation: The needle is shallowly inserted and not retained.

(4) At special acupoint beside the second metacarpal bone:

Location: Lung and heart acupoint.

Method of manipulation: The needle is inserted for 1.6 cm and retained for 10 minutes after mild needling stimulation.

3) Hand *qigong*: Kongjin exercise.

The hand is prone with the palm facing downward and all 10 fingers extended and relaxed. The little finger is flexed downward and then the hands resume the original ladder pattern; all fingers are extended and relaxed and the middle finger is flexed downward and then the hands resume the ladder pattern; then the fingers are extended and relaxed and the little and middle fingers are flexed downward, and the hands resume the ladder pattern. This exercise is repeated 11 times and the entire exercise is ended after a pole-standing exercise in the riding-horse posture for five minutes.

6. Bi-syndrome of chest

This is a group of diseases characterized by distension and pain in the chest radiated to the back, and shortness of breath. Mild cases only feel fullness in the chest, while severe cases may suffer from heart pain radiated to the back and back pain radiated to the heart.

Coronary heart disease, angina pectoris in myocardiac infarction, and precordial pain in pericarditis and other diseases in modern medicine may be treated by the following methods.

Applications of hand therapy:

1) Massage therapy:

Location: Heart area, thumb and middle finger, Shenmen (HT 7), Shaoshang (LU 11), Shaochong (HT 9), Zhongchong (PC 9), lung and heart acupoint and heart reflective point.

Method of manipulation: Kneading and pressing maneuvers applied to the heart area; twisting and pinching at thumb and middle finger; digit-pressing and kneading at Shenmen (HT 7), Shaoshang (LU 11) and Shaochong (HT 9), lung and heart acupoint and heart reflective point.

2) Acupuncture therapy:

(1) At regular and extra acupoint:

Location: Neiguan (PC 6) and Jianshi (PC 5).

Method of manipulation: The needles are inserted to bilateral acupoints for 3.3 cm and retained for 30 minutes after strong stimulation.

(2) At reflective points:

Location: Heart point and chest point.

Method of manipulation: The needles are inserted for 1.6 cm and retained for five minutes.

(3) At reflective areas:

Location: Chest area in palmar reflective areas and radial reverse palmar reflective areas.

Method of manipulation: The needle is shallowly inserted and not retained.

(4) At special acupoint beside the second metacarpal bone:

Location: Lung and heart acupoint.

Method of manipulation: The needle is inserted for 1.6 cm and retained for 20 minutes.

3) Hand bath:

Recipe: Chuanxiong (Rhizoma Ligustici) 60 g, Xiangfu (Rhizoma Cyperi) 30 g, Bingpian (borneol) 5 g, Danshen (Radix Salviae Miltiorhizae) 50 g, and Tanxiang (Lignum Aquilariae) 10 g.

Function: To adjust *qi*, expand chest, promote blood circulation and relieve obstruction.

Method of manipulation: Bingpian is dissolved in a hot decoction of other herbs for steaming and then washing both hands.

4) Hand *qigong*: Physical and breath exercise for distension of chest and abdomen.

The practitioner takes a pole-standing posture with legs separated at shoulder width and heels apart. Breath is adjusted and the mind is stilled. Both arms are crossed and placed on the chest; the slightly flexed legs are still with upper body weight intentionally applied to the lower limbs. The exercise is continued until the distension of chest is released. The effect may be even better if the exercise is continued for a longer time. The attention is concentrated at the navel and the navel *qi* is transported upward through a spiral route to the chest, then to both arms and discharged from Laogong (PC 8) acupoint on both palms. If the distension of chest can be relieved, attention is concentrated at the back and *qi* is transported upward to the head and discharged from Baihui (GV 20) acupoint. This is an effective exercise.

7. Stomachache

This is an ailment with pain of the epigastric area.

Acute and chronic gastritis, peptic ulcer of stomach and

duodenum, cancer of stomach, and gastric neurosis with epigastric pain in modern medicine can be treated by the following methods.

Applications of hand therapy:

1) Massage therapy:

Location: Midline of palm, intestine area, stomach area, spleen area, digestive system, stomach and intestine reflective point, Daling (PC 7), spleen reflective point, duodenum acupoint, forehead reflective point and stomach acupoint.

Method of manipulation: Rubbing maneuver applied at central part of palm, pushing and pressing maneuvers along midline of palm; pressing maneuver at intestine area, stomach area, spleen area, and kidney area; digit-pressing maneuver at stomach and intestine point, Daling (PC 7), stomach acupoint and duodenum acupoint; and pinching and digit-pressing at spleen point and forehead point. A toothpick may be used to press the points and areas; and a burning cigarette may be used to do moxibustion.

2) Acupuncture therapy:

(1) At regular and extra acupoints:

Location: Neiguan (PC 6) and Hegu (LI 4).

Method of manipulation: The needles are vertically inserted for 3.3 cm and retained for 40 minutes after strong stimulation.

(2) At reflective point:

Location: Stomach and intestine point.

Method of manipulation: The needle is inserted for 1.6 cm and retained for five minutes after medium needling stimulation.

(3) At special acupoint beside the second metacarpal bone:

Location: Stomach acupoint.

Method of manipulation: The needle is inserted for 1.6 cm and retained for 15 minutes after strong needling stimulation.

3) Hand bath:

Recipe: Chuanlianzi (Fructus Meliae Toosendan) 20 g, Yanhusuo (Rhizoma Corydalis) 20 g, Wuyao (Radix Linderae) 15 g, Mike (Fructus Papaveris) 10 g, and Honghua (Flos Car-thami) 10 g.

Function: To adjust *qi* and control pain.

Method of manipulation: Routine method to steam and wash both hand.

8. Hiccups

This is a symptom with repeated short noises in the throat due to the adverse ascent of *qi* from below.

In modern medicine, it is believed to be induced by spasms of the diaphragm. Hiccups occur in patients with neuroses of stomach and intestines, gastritis, gastric dilatation, liver cirrho-sis at late stage, cerebrovascular disease, and uremia can all be treated by the following methods.

Applications of hand therapy:

1) Massage therapy:

Location: Laogong (PC 8), Qiangu (SI 2), Zhongkui (EX-UE 4), occipital head reflective point, diaphragm reflective point, stomach acupoint, chest and diaphragm area, and middle finger.

Method of manipulation: Pressing and kneading maneuvers applied at chest and diaphragm area; pushing maneuver from proximal end of middle finger to palm root; pinching and digit-pressing maneuvers at Laogong (PC 8), Qiangu (SI 2), Zhongkui (EX-UE 4), occipital head point and diaphragm point; and kneading maneuver at stomach acupoint. The ma-nipulation should be gently applied. The patients with persistent hiccups, projectile vomiting, and stiff tongue should be trans-ferred to a hospital to rule out cerebrovascular diseases and lesions in the brain.

2) Acupuncture therapy:

(1) At regular and extra acupoints:

Location: Neiguan (PC 6), Zhongkui (EX-UE 4) and Hegu (LI 4).

Method of manipulation: The needles are inserted and re-tained for 30 minutes.

(2) At reflective point:

Location: Hiccup point.

Method of manipulation: The needle is inserted and retained for five minutes.

(3) At special acupoint beside the second metacarpal bone:

Location: Stomach acupoint.

Method of manipulation: The needle is inserted for 1.6 cm and retained for 15 minutes.

3) Hand *qigong*: Physical and breath exercise for vomiting.

The practitioner takes an upright sitting position with both hands extended backward and one wrist held by the other hand. The palm with the wrist held by the other hand is placed on the ground to support the upper body, and the trunk is moved up and down seven times. The exercise is then repeated with the hands reversed. This exercise can treat regurgitation of food and drink due to an attack of wind and cold pathogens and accumulation of *qi* over a long time.

9. Vomiting

According to the theory of traditional Chinese medicine, vomiting is due to the adverse ascent of stomach *qi* and can be divided into two types: One with vomiting without noise, and one with vomiting noise without vomitus. However vomitus and a vomiting noise are usually present together.

Acute gastritis, spasm of cardia, spasm of pylorus, hepatitis, pancreatitis, and cholecystitis with vomiting classified by modern medicine can be treated by the following methods.

Applications of hand therapy:

1) Massage therapy:

Location: Palm, dorsal inter-osseous spaces, Laogong (PC 8), Daling (PC 7), Zhongkui (EX-UE 4), Dagukong (EX-UE 5) and stomach acupoint.

Method of manipulation: Heavy rubbing maneuver applied over palm; pushing maneuver along dorsal inter-osseous spaces; heavy digit-pressing and kneading maneuvers at Laogong (PC 8), Zhongkui (EX-UE 4) and Dagukong (EX-UE 5) acupoints; and digit-pressing maneuver at Daling (PC 7) and stomach acupoint. The heavy manipulation is applied at acute stages of disease.

2) Acupuncture therapy:

(1) At regular and extra acupoints:

Location: Neiguan (PC 6) and Daling (PC 7).

Method of manipulation: The needles are inserted and retained for 30 minutes after medium needling stimulation.

(2) At reflective point:

Location: Chest point.

Method of manipulation: The needle is inserted for one cm and retained for five minutes.

(3) At reflective areas:

Location: Upper abdomen area in palmar reflective areas and ulnar reverse palmar reflective areas.

Method of manipulation: The needle is inserted and then removed right after twisting, lifting, and thrusting stimulation.

(4) At special acupoint beside the second metacarpal bone:

Location: Stomach acupoint.

Method of manipulation: The needle is inserted for 3.3 cm and retained for 20 minutes.

3) Hand *qigong*: Physical and breath exercise for difficult intake of food due to functional disturbance of spleen and stomach.

The patient stands erect with feet apart at a distance the width of the shoulder. The upper body is slightly inclined forward and turned to the left with lower limbs stationary; the dorsum of left hand is held by right palm and also turned to left side; the upper body is stretched with the head and arms turned to right side, and then the upper body is also turned to right side; the body is kept motionless and the body's force and *qi* is held stable for a while; and finally the starting posture with body erect is assumed with the arms freely hanging beside the body. The exercise of both sides may be repeated 21 times (Fig. 41).

4) Herb-holding therapy:

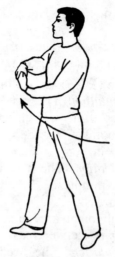

Fig. 41

Herbs: Banxia (pinellia tuber) 10 g and Chenpi (mandarium peel) 12 g.

Method of manipulation: A powder of these herbs is mixed with a paste made of green onion stalks 6 g and fresh ginger 10 g to prepare pills for holding in the palm. If the vomiting cannot be controlled, a decoction of fresh ginger 9 g is orally administered.

10. Dysphagia

In traditional Chinese medicine, dysphagia is divided into two types: In one, food is difficult to swallow, and in the second, food is regurgitated right after intake. Generally, the two types are found together or appear at different stages of a disease.

The dysphagia occurs in cancer of esophagus or cardia, spasms of cardia, esophageal diverticulum, neurosis of esophagus, and esophagitis, all of which may be treated by the following methods.

Applications of hand therapy:

Acupuncture therapy:

(1) At regular and extra acupoints:

Location: Neiguan (PC 6), Hegu (LI 4) and Zhongkui (EX-UE 4).

Method of manipulation: The strong stimulation is applied and the needles are retained for 30 minutes.

(2) At reflective points:

Location: Chest point, stomach, and intestine point.

Method of manipulation: The needles are inserted for 1 cm and retained for five minutes.

(3) At reflective areas:

Location: Chest area and upper abdomen area in palmar reflective areas and ulnar reverse palmar reflective areas.

Method of manipulation: The needles are inserted and removed right after twisting, lifting, and thrusting stimulation.

(4) At special acupoints beside the second metacarpal bone:

Location: Neck acupoint and upper limb acupoint for patients with lesion in esophagus; and stomach acupoint for patients with lesion in stomach.

Method of manipulation: The needles are inserted for 3.3 cm and retained for 15 minutes after medium needling stimulation.

11. Abdominal pain

This is a common symptom with pain in the abdomen below the epigastric region and above the pubic symphysis. It may occur with many diseases, but abdominal pain in dysentery, cholera, abdominal tumors, and intestinal parasites will be discussed later.

Abdominal pain in acute pancreatitis, gastric and intestinal colic, strangulated hernia, gastric and intestinal neurosis, and indigestion classified by modern medicine can all be treated by the following methods.

Applications of hand therapy:

1) Acupuncture therapy:

(1) At regular and extra acupoints:

Location: Quchi (LI 11), Hegu (LI 4) and Neiguan (PC 6).

Method of manipulation: After strong stimulation, the needles are retained for 40 minutes.

(2) At reflective point:

Location: Stomach and intestine point.

Method of manipulation: The needle is shallowly inserted and retained for five minutes after medium needling stimulation.

(3) At reflective area:

Location: Abdomen area in corresponding painful region of palmar reflective areas.

Method of manipulation: The needle is shallowly inserted and not retained.

(4) At special acupoint beside the second metacarpal bone.

Location: The sensitive tender spot between stomach acupoint and leg acupoint.

Method of manipulation: The needle is inserted for 3.3 cm and the strong stimulation is applied.

2) Hand bath:

Recipe: Yanhusuo (Rhizoma Corydalis) 20 g, Wuyao (Radix Linderae) 15 g, Rougui (Saigon Cinnamon) 10 g, dried ginger 15 g, Wuzhuyu (Evodia) 20 g, Xixin (Herba Asari) 3 g, Lizhihe (Semen Litchi) 20 g, and Gancao (Licorice) 10 g.

Function: To warm spleen and stomach, expel cold pathogen, adjust *qi*, and control pain.

Method of manipulation: Routine steaming and washing method for both hands.

3) Hand *qigong*: Physical and breathing exercise for abdominal distension and pain.

The patient assumes a standing position. The body is turned to one side at the utmost range with both arms extended to the same side to move *qi* downward and spread it to both feet; the palm and fingers are extended. The exercise is done on both sides 21 times. The initial standing posture of the body is restored. The shoulders, arms, and waist are rotated back and forth seven times to treat abdominal distension and pain, cold in the urinary bladder, low back and arm pain, and exaggerated pulsation of blood vessels.

12. Dysentery

Dysentery is a disease with symptoms of abdominal pain, tenesmus and diarrhea with blood and pus in stool, and is common in summer and autumn.

Bacillary dysentery in modern medicine can be treated by the following methods.

Applications of hand therapy:

1) Massage therapy:

Location: Stomach area, intestinal area, urinary bladder area, kidney area, dorsal interosseous spaces, Sanjian (LI 3) and diarrhea point.

Method of manipulation: After both palms are rubbed to produce a hot sensation, pressing and kneading maneuvers are applied at the stomach, intestines, urinary bladder, and kidney areas; pushing maneuver along dorsal interosseous spaces toward fingers, and continuous digit-pressing and kneading maneuvers at Sanjian (LI 3) and diarrhea point.

2) Acupuncture therapy:

(1) At regular and extra acupoints:

Location: Quchi (LI 11) and Hegu (LI 4) acupoints.

Method of manipulation: After strong stimulation, the needles are retained for 30 minutes.

(2) At reflective point:

Location: Stomach point.

Method of manipulation: The needle is inserted for 1 cm and retained for five minutes.

(3) At special acupoint beside the second metacarpal bone:

Location: Sensitive tender spot between stomach acupoint and leg acupoint.

Method: The needle is inserted for 1.6 cm and retained for 30 minutes after medium needling stimulation.

13. Diarrhea

In patients with diarrhea, a loose or watery stool may be frequently passed due to diseases of the spleen, stomach or large and small intestines. It may occur anytime, but is most common in summer and autumn.

Acute and chronic enteritis, tuberculosis of the intestines, dysfunction of intestines, and irritable colon with diarrhea can be treated by the following methods.

Applications of hand therapy:

1) Massage therapy:

Location: Chest reflective point, stomach and intestine reflective point, chest and abdomen area, Sanjian (LI 3), diarrhea point, Dagukong (EX-UE 5), stomach acupoint, stomach area, intestine area, liver area, large intestine acupoint and kidney acupoint.

Method of manipulation: Digit-pressing and kneading maneuvers applied at stomach area, digestive tract area, intestine area and anus area; pressing and kneading maneuvers at chest reflective point, stomach and intestine reflective point, Sanjian (LI 3), diarrhea point, Dagukong (EX-UE 5) and stomach acupoint; and pinching and digit-pressing maneuvers at large intestine acupoint and kidney acupoint.

2) Acupuncture therapy:

(1) At regular and extra acupoints:

Location: Quchi (LI 11), Hegu (LI 4) and Shousanli (LI 10).

Method of manipulation: The needles are inserted and retained for 30 minutes.

(2) At reflective points:

Location: Stomach and intestine point and spleen point.

Method of manipulation: The needles are inserted for 1.6 cm and retained for three minutes.

(3) At special acupoint beside the second metacarpal bone:

Location: Sensitive tender spot between stomach acupoint and leg acupoint.

Method of manipulation: The needle is inserted for 3.3 cm and retained for 20 minutes.

3) Hand bath:

Recipe: Mike (Fructus Papaeris) 20 g, Roudoukou (Semen Myrisiticae) 20 g, Guizhi (cassia twig) 20 g, Wuzhuyu (Evodiae) 30 g, Muxiang (costus root) 20 g and Chenpi (mandarium peel) 20 g.

Function: To warm spleen and stomach and stop diarrhea.

Method of manipulation: A hot decoction of these herbs is used to steam and then wash both hands for 30 minutes, two to three times a day.

14. Constipation

This is a disease characterized by hard stools difficult to pass, and prolonged intervals between bowel movements.

Habitual constipation, reduced strength of bowel movements due to general weakness, reduced intestinal peristalsis in recovery stage of enteritis, anal fissure, hemorrhoids, and proctitis in modern medicine can be treated by the following methods.

Applications of hand therapy

1) Massage therapy:

Location: Central part of palm, proximal ends of finger and web border between fingers, Erjian (LI 2), Sanjian (LI 3), Hegu (LI 4), intestine area, anus area, and digestive tract.

Method of manipulation: Grinding and pushing maneuvers applied at intestine area, anus area, and digestive tract; pinching and kneading maneuvers at proximal ends of fingers and web border between fingers; and digit-pressing and kneading maneuvers at Erjian (LI 2), Sanjian (LI 3) and Hegu (LI 4) acupoints. Pressing maneuver is applied at head area and adrenal gland area for treating habitual constipation; and pressing maneuver at kidney area for senile constipation. The manipulation should be persistently and gently applied.

2) Acupuncture therapy:

(1) At regular and extra acupoints:

Location: Zhigou (TE 6) and Hegu (LI 4).

Method of manipulation: The needles are vertically inserted for 3.3 cm and retained for 30 minutes.

(2) At special acupoints beside the second metacarpal bone:

Location: Kidney acupoint and lower abdomen acupoint.

Method of manipulation: The needles are inserted for 2.6 cm

and retained for 15 minutes.

3) Herb-holding therapy:

Herbs: Roucongrong (Herba Cistanches) 15 g and sulfur 6 g.

Method of manipulation: After these herbs are pounded into small bits, one half of the pounded herbs is held in palms and the other half applied over the navel to treat constipation due to deficiency of *yang*.

15. Costal pain

According to traditional Chinese medicine, the liver lies in the costal region with the gallbladder attached to liver, and their meridians also pass through the costal region. Therefore, costal pain is closely related to the liver and gallbladder.

Acute and chronic hepatitis, liver cirrhosis, parasites of the liver, liver abscess, liver cancer, acute and chronic cholecystitis, ascaris in biliary tract, and costal neuralgia with costal pain can be treated by the following methods.

Applications of hand therapy

1) Acupuncture therapy:

(1) At regular and extra acupoints:

Location: Waiguan (TE 5), Zhongdu (TE 3), Zhigou (TE 6) and Wangu (SI 4).

Method of manipulation: The needles are inserted and retained for 30 minutes after strong needling stimulation.

(2) At reflective point:

Location: Temporal head reflective point.

Method of manipulation: The needle is inserted for 1.6 cm and retained for five minutes.

(3) At special acupoint beside the second metacarpal bone:

Location: Liver acupoint.

Method of manipulation: The needle is inserted for 1.6 cm and retained for 30 minutes.

2) Hand *qigong*:

(1) Physical and breathing exercises for liver diseases.

The patient assumes a straight sitting posture or sits with legs crossed and with both hands in front of the chest with fingers separated as though holding a ball. The distance between the hands is 10 cm, and between hands and chest, 20 cm. The chest is drawn in with back straightened, and the shoulders and elbows drooped with the armpits opened. The hands are horizontally drawn apart to chest width, and then drawn close together to the original distance between them. This drawing hands exercise is repeated several times. The palms are turned inward to face the chest, making circles five to six times (Fig. 42) within a range between Danzhong (CV 17) and Guanyuan (CV 4) acupoints.

(2) Kongjin hand exercise:

The hand is prone with the palm facing downward to flex the middle and ring fingers (Fig. 43) and then to resume the original hand ladder pattern. The finger exercise is repeated nine times and the whole set of exercises is ended after a pole-standing exercise in the riding posture for five minutes.

16. Abdominal mass

This is a disease whose symptoms include abdominal mass, pain, and distension.

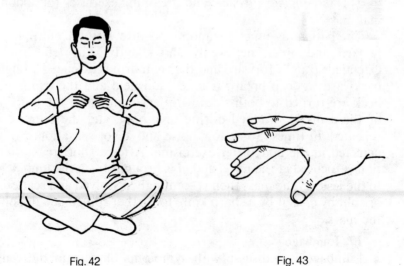

Fig. 42   Fig. 43

Abdominal tumors, enlargement of the liver and spleen, stomach dysfunction and intestinal obstruction in modern medicine can be treated by the following methods.

Applications of hand therapy:

1) Acupuncture therapy:

(1) At regular and extra acupoints:

Location: Quchi (LI 11), Shousanli (LI 10) and Hegu (LI 4).

Method of manipulation: The needles are inserted and retained for 30 minutes.

(2) At reflective points:

Location: Stomach and intestine point and triple energizer point.

Method of manipulation: The needles are inserted for 1 cm and retained for five minutes.

(3) At special acupoint beside the second metacarpal bone:

Location: Stomach acupoint or sensitive tender spot between stomach acupoint and leg acupoint.

Method of manipulation: The needle is inserted for 1.6 cm and retained for 20 minutes.

2) Hand *qigong*: Physical and breathing exercises for abdominal mass.

The patient assumes a standing posture with the entire body relaxed and breathing evenly and silently. The left arm is extended straight forward and the right arm is extended straight backward; a deep breath is taken and held and the trunk and neck are turned to both sides with legs stationary; the position of the arms is switched during breathing, and the exercise is repeated 70 times. Some low noise and a hot sensation can be detected in the body after exercising. After a short rest, attention is focused at the navel and *qi* is brought from the umbilicus to the lesion. The mass then is seemingly dissolved and scattered or split by *qi* as if by a sharp knife to further spread and dissolve the mass.

17. Lumbago

Lumbago is a disease with symptoms of pain in the waist

area and which may occur on one or both sides of the body.

The lumbago in diseases of spinal column, injury of soft tissues beside spinal column, compression of spinal nerve roots or other medical and gynecological diseases may be treated by the following methods.

Applications of hand therapy:

1) Acupuncture therapy:

(1) At regular and extra acupoints:

Location: Yanglao (SI 6) and Houxi (SI 3).

Method of manipulation: The strong stimulation is applied with local massage.

(2) At reflective point:

Location: Waist reflective point.

Method of manipulation: The needle is inserted for 1.6 cm and retained for five minutes after strong needling stimulation.

(3) At reflective areas:

Location: Waist area in dorsal reflective areas and radial or ulnar reverse dorsal reflective areas.

Method of manipulation: After twisting, lifting and thrusting stimulation, the needles are immediately removed.

(4) At special acupoint beside the second metacarpal bone:

Location: Waist acupoint.

Method of manipulation: The needle is inserted for 3.3 cm and retained for 30 minutes.

2) Hand *qigong*:

The patient assumes a standing position with one leg thrust forward and the entire body relaxed with the breath quiescent. The arm on the side with leg forward is raised up to the limit with the palm turned upward; then the arm is rotated with the fingers turned; the other hand is pressed downward with palm facing backward. The forward leg is moved back, the palms placed together and, following the upper body, they are turned to one side with the eyes focused on them. The *qi* is intentionally moved downward, and then upward after it is dispersed throughout the lower body. This exercise is repeated on both sides 28 times to relieve the dull pain over the shoulder, costal region, and lumbar spinal column (Figs. 44 and 45).

18. Retention of urine

This is a disease with reduced discharge or complete cessation of urination; the former condition is called "long" and the latter condition is called "bi" in traditional Chinese medicine.

The retention of urine and urea in modern medicine can be treated by the following methods.

Applications of hand therapy:

1) Acupuncture therapy:

(1) At regular and extra acupoints:

Location: Shaoshang (LU 11) and Hegu (LI 4) acupoints.

Method of manipulation: Bleeding therapy with three-edged needle is applied at Shaoshang (LU 11), and the regular needle is punctured at Hegu (LI 4) acupoint for 3.3 cm and retained for 30 minutes.

(2) At reflective areas:

Location: Perineum area of palmar reflective areas and ulnar or radial reverse palmar reflective areas.

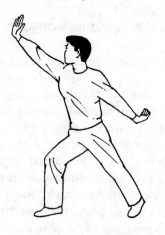
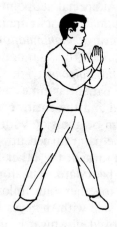

Fig. 44   Fig. 45

Method of manipulation: The needles are shallowly inserted and removed right after the twisting, lifting, and thrusting stimulation.

(3) At special acupoint beside the second metacarpal bone:
Location: Lower abdomen acupoint.
Method of manipulation: The needle is inserted for 1.6 cm and retained for 15 minutes after medium needling stimulation.

2) Hand bath:
Recipe: Taozhi (Ramulus Persicae), Liuzhi (Ramulus Salicis), Mutong (Caulis Aristolochiae Manshuriensis), Huajiao (Pericarpium Zanthoxyli), and Mingfan (Alumen) 30 g of each, fresh green onion stalks 100 g and Dengxin (Medulla Junci) 15 g.

Function: To promote discharge of urine and relieve dribbling urination.

Method of manipulation: The herbs are wrapped in gauze and boiled in water to prepare a hot decoction for steaming and washing both hands and perineal region for 30-40 minutes, twice a day.

19. Incontinence of urine

In traditional Chinese medicine this disease is divided into two types: The spontaneous discharge of urine at night stops in the morning; and incontinence of urine out of control during the day.

Incontinence of urine and bed-wetting in children and adults due to dysfunction of nervous system or diseases of urinary system can be treated by the following methods.

1) Acupuncture therapy:
(1) At reflective point:
Location: Bed-wetting point.
Method of manipulation: The needle is inserted for 1.6 cm and retained for three minutes.

(2) At reflective areas:
Location: Perineum area in palmar reflective areas and ulnar reverse palmar reflective areas.

Method of manipulation: The needles are shallowly inserted and removed right after twisting, lifting, and thrusting stimulation.

(3) At special acupoint beside the second metacarpal bone:

Location: Lower abdomen acupoint.

Method of manipulation: The needle is inserted for 1.6 cm and retained for 20 minutes.

2) Hand bath:

Recipe: Yizhiren (Semen Alpiniae Oxyphyllae) 20 g, Sangpiaoxiao (Ootheca Mantidis) 30 g, Longgu (fossil bone) 30 g, and Shanzhuyu (Fructus Corni) 20 g.

Function: To tone kidney and control incontinence of urine.

Method of manipulation: A hot decoction of these herbs is used to steam and then wash both hands for 30 minutes, two to three times a day.

20. Emission of semen

This is the discharge of semen without sexual intercourse. In traditional Chinese medicine, it is divided into two types: The emission of semen with dreams of sexual activity at night; and discharge of semen without dreams and even with a clear mind.

The spontaneous discharge of semen in patients with neurasthenia, prostatitis and seminal vesiculitis can be treated by the following methods.

Applications of hand therapy:

1) Massage therapy:

Location: Palm and dorsum of hand, kidney area, reproductive area, and bed-wetting point.

Method of manipulation: Both hands, especially the palm and dorsum, are rubbed to produce a hot sensation; heavy digit-pressing maneuver applied at kidney and reproductive areas; persistent digit-pressing and kneading maneuvers at bed-wetting point.

2) Acupuncture therapy:

(1) At reflective point:

Location: Kidney point.

Method of manipulation: The needle is inserted for 1.6 cm and retained for five minutes.

(2) At reflective areas:

Location: Perineum area in palmar reflective areas and ulnar reverse palmar reflective areas.

Method of manipulation: The needle is shallowly inserted and immediately removed after needling stimulation.

(3) At special acupoints beside the second metacarpal bone:

Location: Kidney acupoint and lower abdomen acupoint.

Method of manipulation: The needles are inserted for 1.6 cm and retained for 20 minutes.

3) Hand bath:

Recipe: Sangpiaoxiao (Ootheca Mantidis) 30 g, Yuanzhi (Radix Polygalae) 30 g, Longgu (fossil bone) 30 g, Danggui (Chinese Angelica) 30 g, Guiban (Plastrum Testudinis) 20 g, Fuling (Poris cocos) 30 g, and Dangshen (Radix Codonopsis) 30 g.

Function: To adjust and tone heart and kidney and control spontaneous discharge of semen.

Method of manipulation: A hot decoction of these herbs is used to steam and then wash both hands for 20-30 minutes, twice a day.

4) Hand *qigong*: Kongjin exercise.

The hand is prone with palm facing downward and with the fingers kept in the ladder pattern. The ring and little fingers are flexed for 15 minutes, and then the middle finger is also flexed for 10 more minutes or longer for better results. The flexed fingers should not be extended before the exercise is ended by making hollow fists.

5) Herb-holding therapy:

Herbs: Pixiao (Sodium Sulfate) 60 g.

Method of manipulation: The Pixiao is held in both palms until it is completely dissolved, twice a day.

21. Impotence

Impotence is the poor or failed erection of the penis for

sexual intercourse.

Impotence in patients with sexual disorders or other chronic diseases can be treated by the following methods.

Applications of hand therapy:

1) Massage therapy:

Location: Kidney area, reproductive area, reproductive gland area, both little fingers, and Mingmen (life gate) point.

Method of manipulation: The hands are rubbed to produce a hot sensation. Persistent pressing and kneading maneuvers applied at kidney area, reproductive area, reproductive gland area and kidney reflective point; pinching maneuver at Mingmen point; and twisting and rotating both little fingers.

2) Acupuncture therapy: Same as that for emission of semen.

3) Hand bath:

Recipe: Duzhong (Cortex Eucommiae) 50 g, Sangjisheng (Ramulus Loranthi) 30 g, Gouqizi (Fructus Lycii) 30 g, Suoyang (Herba Cynomorii) 30 g, Guizhi (cassia twig) 30 g, Yinyanghuo (Herba Epimedii) 30 g, and Tusizi (Semen Cuscutae) 30 g.

Function: To warm and tone kidney *yang*, essence, and blood.

Method of manipulation: A hot decoction of these herbs is used to steam and then wash both hands for 30 minutes, twice a day.

4) Hand *qigong*: Physical and breathing exercise for kidney diseases.

The patient assumes a straight sitting position or sitting with legs crossed posture with eyes closed and the breath quiescent. Both arms are raised to the ears fully extended, and then drooped down until freely hanging beside the thighs, three to five times. The right hand is raised from the side of thigh to chest level and swayed to the right side as if throwing an object, and this movement is then repeated on the left side. This exercise of swaying arms to both sides is repeated several times.

22. Insomnia

This is a disease of disturbed sleep. In mild insomnia, the

patient may have difficulty falling asleep, is easily awakened, and finds it difficult to go back to sleep once awakened. In cases of severe insomnia, the patient cannot fall asleep all night.

Insomnia in patients with neurasthenia, hypertension, cerebral arteriosclerosis, anemia, hepatitis, menopausal syndrome, and psychoneurosis in modern medicine can be treated by the following methods.

Applications of hand therapy:

1) Massage therapy:

Location: Head area, insomnia area, Shenmen (HT 7) and Zhongchong (PC 9).

Method of manipulation: Both hands are rubbed to produce a hot sensation. Heavy pushing and rubbing maneuvers are applied to palm, and a pushing maneuver along radial and ulnar borders of fingers and continuous pinching, digit-pressing and kneading maneuvers at Shenmen and palmar surface of fingers; digit-pressing and kneading maneuvers at head area and insomnia area; digit-pressing maneuver with nail at Zhongchong; and rotating and pulling fingers. Each manipulation is repeated 30-50 times.

2) Acupuncture therapy:

(1) At regular and extra acupoints:

Location: Neiguan (PC 6) and Shenmen (HT 7) acupoints.

Method of manipulation: The needles are inserted and retained for 30 minutes.

(2) At reflective point:

Location: Heart point.

Method of manipulation: The needle is inserted for 1.6 cm and retained for five minutes.

(3) At special acupoints beside the second metacarpal bone:

Location: Head acupoint, and lung and heart acupoint.

Method of manipulation: The needles are inserted for 1.6 cm and retained for 20 minutes.

3) Hand bath:

Recipe: Cishi (Magnetitum) 50 g, Suanzaoren (Semen Zizyphi Spinosae) 30 g, Baiziren (Arbor Vitae) 30 g, Danggui (Chinese Angelica) 20 g, Zhimu (Rhizoma Anemarrhenae) 10 g, and Yejiaoteng (Caulis Polygoni Multiflori) 30 g.

Function: To tranquilize the mind.

Method of manipulation: A hot decoction of these herbs is used to steam and then wash both hands for 30 minutes, once every night before going to bed.

4) Hand *qigong*: Kongjin exercise.

The hand is prone with palm facing downward and the fingers relaxed. The thumb, ring finger, and little finger are flexed 11 times, and after each repetition the hand resumes a ladder pattern. The index finger is extended upward and then flexed downward twice, then the hand again resumes the ladder pattern. The exercise is ended after a pole-standing exercise in a riding posture for five minutes.

23. Diabetes mellitus

The symptoms of this disease are excessive thirst, overeating, polyuria, pathological leanness, and sweet, turbid urine.

Applications of hand therapy:

1) Massage therapy:

Location: Throat, mouth, esophagus, stomach, and kidney areas, midline of palm, Taiyuan (LU 9), Daling (PC 7), endocrine area, stomach and intestine reflective point, heel reflective point, and Yangchi (TE 4) acupoint.

Method of manipulation: Both hands are rubbed to produce a hot sensation. Heavy pressing, kneading and pinching maneuvers repeatedly applied along midline of palm; continuous digit-pressing maneuver at Taiyuan (LU 9), Daling (PC 7), endocrine area, stomach and intestine point, heel point, and Yangchi (TE 4) in sequence.

2) Acupuncture therapy:

(1) At regular and extra acupoints:

Location: Yangchi (TE 4), Zhizheng (SI 7) and Yuji (LU 10) acupoints.

Method of manipulation: The needles are vertically inserted for 1.6 cm and retained for 30 minutes.

(2) At reflective points:

Location: Lung point, spleen point, and kidney point.

Method of manipulation: The needles are inserted for 1.6 cm and retained for five minutes after twisting, lifting, and thrusting stimulation.

(3) At special acupoints beside the second metacarpal bone:

Location: Lung and heart acupoint, stomach acupoint, and kidney acupoint.

Method of manipulation: The needles are vertically inserted for 1.6 cm and retained for 20 minutes.

24. Vertigo

Vertigo is called *xuanyun* in traditional Chinese medicine, since the blurred vision is called *xuan* and dizziness is called *yun*. In mild cases, the symptoms may disappear when the eyes are closed; in severe cases, patients may suffer from nausea, vomiting, sweating, difficulty standing, symptoms of motion sickness, and even syncope.

Auditory vertigo, cerebral vertigo, toxic vertigo and vertigo in patients with paroxysmal tachycardia, auriculoventricular blockage, anemia, cerebral injury, and neurasthenia can be treated by the following methods.

Applications of hand therapy:

1) Massage therapy:

Location: Guanchong (TE 1) and Zhongchong (PC 9) acupoints.

Method of manipulation: Pinching maneuver is applied at Guanchong and Zhongchong acupoints by nail.

2) Acupuncture therapy:

(1) At regular and extra acupoints:

Location: Neiguan (PC 6) and Hegu (LI 4) acupoints.

Method of manipulation: The needles are vertically inserted for 3.3 cm and retained for 30 minutes.

(2) At reflective areas:

Location: Head area in dorsal reflective areas and radial or ulnar reverse dorsal reflective areas.

Method of manipulation: The needles are shallowly inserted and immediately removed after twisting, lifting, and thrusting stimulation.

(3) At special acupoints beside the second metacarpal bone:

Location: Head acupoint, and kidney acupoint in vertigo caused by kidney deficiency.

Method of manipulation: The needles are inserted for 1.6 cm and retained for 30 minutes.

3) Hand bath:

Recipe: Wuzhuyu (Evodia) 10 g, Yejiaoteng (Caulis Polygoni Multiflori) 20 g, Muli (Concha Ostreae) 30 g, Luobuma (Herba Apocyni) 15 g, and Xijiancao (Herba Siegesbeckiae) 10 g.

Function: To suppress liver *yang* and tranquilize the mind.

Method of manipulation: A hot decoction of the above herbs is used to steam and then wash both hands for 20-30 minutes, two to three times a day to treat vertigo due to hypertension with an upward disturbance of liver *yang*.

4) Hand *qigong*: Kongjin exercise.

The hand is prone with palm facing downward and the fingers relaxed. The ring and little fingers are simultaneously flexed at the interphalangeal joint with finger tips pointing downward (Fig. 46) and the hands assuming the original ladder pattern with the fingers relaxed and extended; the ring and little fingers are then flexed at the metacarpophalangeal joint (Fig. 47) and the hands resume the ladder pattern. This exercise is repeated six times and then ended after a pole-standing exercise in a riding posture for five minutes to treat vertigo due to hypertension (an upward disturbance of liver *yang*).

25. Cerebral apoplexy

Cerebral apoplexy is also called stroke with symptoms of collapse, loss of consciousness, deviation of mouth and eye, hemiplegia and aphasia, or with clear consciousness and deviation of mouth and eye, and hemiplegia alone.

The hemorrhagic and ischemic cerebrovascular diseases in

modern medicine can be treated by the following methods.

Applications of hand therapy:

1) Massage therapy:

Location: Head area, pads and joints of fingers, Shenmen (HT 7), Shaoshang (LU 11), Erjian (LI 2), Hegu (LI 4), Shaoze (SI 1) and Qiangu (SI 2) acupoints.

Method of manipulation: Continuous digit-pressing and kneading maneuvers applied to head area; pinching and kneading maneuvers at radial and ulnar borders and pads of fingers; twisting and pulling joints of fingers; heavy digit-pressing and pinching maneuvers at Shenmen (HT 7), Shaoshang (LU 11), Erjian (LI 2), Hegu (LI 4), Shaozi (SI 1) and Qiangu (SI 2) acupoints, especially heavy manipulation applied to the affected side; and pinching maneuver at nail beds.

2) Acupuncture therapy:

(1) At regular and extra acupoints:

Location: In patients with attack at internal organs, 12 *Jing* points and Shixuan (EX-UE 11) are selected; in patients with attack at meridians, the location is determined according to clinical manifestations; in patients with speech disturbance, Tongli (HT 5), Neiguan (PC 6) and Hegu (LI 4) are used; in patients with numbness and paralysis of upper limbs, Quchi (LI

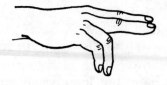

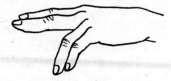

Fig. 46   Fig. 47

11), Waiguan (TE 5) and Hegu are used; and in patients with damage to lower limbs, Quchi (LI 11) and Houxi (SI 3) of the contralateral side are used. Patients are asked to move the affected limbs during the application of acupuncture.

Method of manipulation: Bleeding therapy with three-edged needle is applied at 12 *Jing* points and Shixuan (EX-UE 11) and routine acupuncture is applied at other points.

(2) At reflective areas:

Location: The location is determined according to the location of the lesion. For example, the right upper limb area in dorsal reflective areas and radial reverse dorsal reflective areas may be selected.

Method of manipulation: The needle is shallowly inserted for application of medium needling stimulation.

(3) At special acupoints beside the second metacarpal bone:

Location: Head acupoint and corresponding acupoints of the affected limbs. For example, in patients with paralysis of upper limb, the head acupoint and upper limb acupoint are used.

Method of manipulation: The needles are inserted for 1.6 cm for application of strong stimulation.

26. Muscular atrophy

This is a disease with flaccidity and weakness of muscles, and sometimes complete muscular atrophy.

Muscular atrophy in multiple neuritis, acute myelitis, and progressive myotrophy in modern medicine can be treated by the following methods.

Applications of hand therapy:

1) Acupuncture therapy:

(1) At regular and extra acupoints:

Location: Quchi (LI 11), Waiguan (TE 5), Shousanli (LI 10) and Hegu (LI 4) acupoints.

Method of manipulation: The needles are inserted and retained for 30 minutes.

(2) At reflective areas:

Location: The reflective areas of the affected limbs in dorsal reflective areas and ulnar or radial reverse dorsal reflective areas.

Method of manipulation: The needles are shallowly inserted, but not retained.

(3) At special acupoints beside the second metacarpal bone:

Location: The location is determined according to the location of the lesion. For example, in injury to upper limb, the upper limb acupoint is used; and in injury to lower limb, the lower limb acupoint is used.

Method of manipulation: The needles are inserted for 1.6 cm and retained for 30 minutes after strong needling stimulation.

2) Hand bath:

Recipe: Huangbo (Cortex Phellodendri) 150 g, Guiban (Plastrum Testudinis) 120 g, Zhimu (Rhizoma Anemarrhenae) 30 g, Chenpi (mandarium peel) 60 g, Baishao (white peony), Suoyang (Herba Cynomorii) 30 g, Gusuibu (Rhizoma Drynariae) 20 g, and dried ginger 30 g.

Function: To tone *yin*, suppress fire pathogen, and strengthen muscle and bone.

Method of manipulation: A hot decoction of these herbs is used to steam and then wash both hands for 30 minutes, twice a day. It is best to do a foot bath at the same time.

27. Epilepsy

This is a disease with paroxysmal attacks of mental confusion, sudden collapse, loss of consciousness, foaming at the mouth, upward staring of eyes and convulsion of limbs with noise cried from mouth. The patients may restore their consciousness after the attack.

This is similar to primary or secondary epilepsy in modern medicine and can be treated by the following methods.

Applications of hand therapy:

1) Massage therapy:

Location: Shenmen (HT 7), Laogong (PC 8), chest reflective point, palm and dorsum of hand, Hegu (LI 4), Houxi (SI 3), Yanggu (SI 5) and Shixuan (EX-UE 11).

Method of manipulation: The palm and dorsum of the hands are rubbed and pushed to produce a hot sensation; pinching maneuver applied at Shenmen (HT 7), Laogong (PC 8), chest reflective point, Hegu (LI 4), Houxi (SI 3), Yanggu (SI 5) and Shixuan (EX-UE 11); and digit-pressing maneuver with nail over palmar side of fingers. During attack, digit-pressing and pinching maneuvers are applied at head area and head reflective point.

2) Acupuncture therapy:

(1) At regular and extra acupoints:

Location: Neiguan (PC 6), Hegu (LI 4) and Laogong (PC 8) acupoints.

Method of manipulation: The needles are inserted for 3.3 cm and retained for 30 minutes after strong needling stimulation.

(2) At reflective points:

Location: Heart point and liver point.

Method of manipulation: The needles are inserted for 1.3 cm and retained for five minutes after twisting, lifting, and thrusting stimulation.

(3) At special acupoints beside the second metacarpal bone:

Location: Head acupoint, lung and heart acupoint, and liver acupoint.

Method of manipulation: The needles are inserted for 1.6 cm and retained for 30 minutes.

3) Hand *qigong*: Physical and breath exercise for epilepsy.

During an attack, the patient's wrist is held tightly in the doctor's hand with his thumb forcibly pressing Neiguan and the middle finger of the patient is held in the doctor's other hand with his nail pinching the tip of patient's middle finger (the terminal of pericardium meridian) to resolve the accumulated phlegm (Fig. 48). After consciousness is restored, symptoms relieved, and emotional stability recovered, the patient is taught to relax his body, adjust breathing, become quiescent, and concentrate his attention at the navel to intentionally resolve the accumulated phlegm and move it downward from both sides of

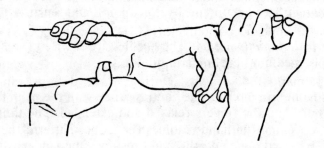

Fig. 48

the heart into the intestine to be discharged from the anus.

28. Psychosis

This is a psychiatric disease which is divided into two types in traditional Chinese medicine: The Dian-syndrome is characterized by an apathetic expression, silence, mental dullness, speaking nonsense, and diminished motion; and the Kuang-syndrome is characterized by mental excitement, hyper-irritability, restlessness, noise making, beating and scolding others, destruction and extreme fury.

The psychiatric diseases of modern medicine are similar to this disease and can be treated by the following methods.

Applications of hand therapy:

1) Acupuncture therapy:

(1) At regular and extra acupoints:

Location: Shaoshang (LU 11), Shaochong (HT 9), Zhong-chong (PC 9) and Guanchong (TE 1) acupoints.

Method of manipulation: The acupoints are punctured by regular acupuncture needles.

(2) At reflective points:

Location: Heart point, lung point, spleen point, and liver point.

Method of manipulation: The points are punctured by regular acupuncture needles.

(3) At special acupoints beside the second metacarpal bone:

Location: Head acupoint, liver acupoint, and sensitive tender spots.

Method of manipulation: The needles are inserted for 1.6 cm to apply medium needling stimulation.

2) Hand *qigong*:

(1) Kongjin exercise: The hand is prone with the palm facing downward and the fingers relaxed and extended. The thumb is flexed once and the hand resumes the ladder pattern; the little finger is flexed once and the hand resumes the ladder pattern; and the index finger is slightly dorsally extended and then flexed once. The exercise of three fingers in sequence is repeated six times and is ended after a pole-standing exercise in riding posture for five minutes.

(2) Physical and breath exercise for psychosis: Same as those for epilepsy.

29. Dementia

This is a neurological disease with mental dullness, apathetic expression, silence, no desire to speak, and poor memory. Severely affected patients cannot take care of their daily needs and are in danger of injuring themselves.

Congenital and senile dementia and dementia following psychosis in modern medicine can be treated by the following methods.

Applications of hand therapy:

1) Acupuncture therapy:

(1) At regular and extra acupoints:

Location: Neiguan (PC 6), Shenmen (HT 7) and Hegu (LI 4) acupoints.

Method of manipulation: The acupoints are punctured by regular needles.

(2) At reflective points:

Location: Heart point and kidney point.

Method of manipulation: The needles are vertically inserted for 1.6 cm and retained for five minutes.

(3) At reflective areas:

Location: Heart area and head area in palmar reflective areas and ulnar or radial reverse palmar reflective areas.

Method of manipulation: The needles are shallowly inserted, but not retained.

(4) At special acupoints beside the second metacarpal bone:

Location: Head acupoint, lung and heart acupoint, and kidney acupoint.

Method of manipulation: The needles are inserted for 1.6 cm and retained for 15 minutes.

30. Shock

The major symptoms of this disease are sudden collapse, loss of consciousness, and cold limbs. In mild cases, the period of unconsciousness is short and the patient does not develop hemiplegia, aphasia, or deviation of mouth and eye after recovering consciousness.

Heat stroke, hypoglycemia, coma, and psychiatric disorders are all related to shock and can be treated by the following methods.

Applications of hand therapy:

1) Acupuncture therapy:

(1) At regular and extra acupoints:

Location: Neiguan (PC 6), Hegu (LI 4) and Laogong (PC 8) acupoints.

Method of manipulation: The needles are inserted and retained for 20 minutes.

(2) At reflective points:

Location: Heart point and liver point.

Method of manipulation: The needles are inserted for 1.6 cm and retained for five minutes.

31. Bi-syndrome

This is a disease with pain, numbness, heaviness, limited movement, and sometimes swollen joints.

Rheumatic fever, rheumatic arthritis, rheumatoid arthritis, and neuralgia sciatica are included under this disease and can be treated by the following methods.

Applications of hand therapy:

1) Massage therapy:

Location: Joints of finger and wrist, palmar and dorsal interosseous spaces, Hegu (LI 4), Yangxi (LI 5), Yangchi (TE 4), waist and leg reflective point, outer Laogong (EX-UE 8) and forehead reflective point.

Method of manipulation: Pressing and kneading maneuvers applied at joints of fingers and wrist; heavy pressing maneuver along palmar and dorsal interosseous spaces; twisting, pulling and rotating joints of fingers and wrist; and pressing and kneading maneuvers at Hegu (LI 4), Yangxi (LI 5), Yangchi (TE 4), waist and leg reflective point, outer Laogong (EX-UE 8) and forehead reflective point.

2) Acupuncture therapy:

(1) At reflective points:

Location: The location for manipulation is determined by the location of the pain. For example, the shoulder point is used for shoulder pain; the spine point for spinal column pain; the sciatic nerve point for neuralgia sciatica; and the neck point is for neck and nape pain.

Method of manipulation: The needles are inserted for 1.3 cm and retained for 20 minutes after medium needling stimulation.

(2) At reflective areas:

Location: The region corresponding to the area of pain in dorsal reflective areas and radial or ulnar reverse dorsal reflective areas.

Method of manipulation: The needles are shallowly inserted and removed immediately after strong needling stimulation.

(3) At special acupoints beside the second metacarpal bone:

Location: According to the location of the pain. For example, the neck acupoint is used for neck pain, and the leg acupoint for leg pain.

3) Hand bath:

Recipe: Chuanwu (Radix Aconiti) 15 g, Caowu (Jack-in-the-

Pulpit) 15 g, Tougucao (Herba Speranskiae) 30 g, Jianghuang (Rhizoma Curcumae Longae) 20 g, Haitongpi (Cortex Erthrinae) 15 g, Weilingxian (Chinese Clematis) 15 g, Sumu (Lignum Sappan) 15 g, Wujiapi (Cortex Acanthopanacis Radicis) 15 g, and Honghua (Flos Carthami) 10 g.

Function: To promote blood circulation, release stagnant blood, expel wind and cold pathogens, resolve dampness, and stop pain.

Method of manipulation: A hot decoction of these herbs is used to steam and then wash both hands and painful area for 30 minutes, two to three times a day.

4) Hand *qigong*: Physical and breath exercise for pain of Bi-syndrome.

The patient sits upright and raises the right hand with the palm facing upward and covered by left arm. The left hand is slightly shaken with the intake of nasal breath. This is repeated seven times to relieve pain of both arms and the back.

32. Numbness

This is a disease with numbness and even loss of sensation in skin, muscles, and limbs.

The numbness of skin and muscles in various diseases of connective tissue, and nutritional, metabolic, and endocranial diseases can be treated by the following methods.

Applications of hand therapy:

1) Acupuncture therapy:

(1) At regular and extra acupoints:

Location: The location of acupuncture is determined by the location of the lesion. For example, Quchi (LI 11), Hegu (LI 4) and Waiguan (TE 5) are used for numbness of the upper limbs; Baxie (EX-UE 9), Houxi (TE 3), Neiguan (PC 6) and Hegu for numbness of the hands; and Shixuan (EX-UE 11) for numbness of the fingers.

Method of manipulation: Bleeding therapy is applied at Shixuan, and routine acupuncture is applied at other acupoints after retention of needles for 20 minutes.

(2) At reflective areas:

Location: Areas corresponding to the region of numbness in dorsal reflective areas and radial or ulnar reverse dorsal reflective areas.

Method of manipulation: The needles are shallowly inserted and removed immediately after twisting, lifting, and thrusting stimulation.

(3) At special acupoints beside the second metacarpal bone:

Location: According to the area of numbness. For example, the upper limb acupoint is used for numbness of the upper limbs; and the leg acupoint is used for lower limb numbness.

Method of manipulation: Routine manipulation.

2) Hand bath:

Recipe: Sangzhi (Ramulus Mori) 30 g, Guizhi (cassia twig) 20 g, Weilingxian (Chinese Clematis) 15 g, Xijiancao (Herba Siegesbeckiae) 30 g, 2 pieces of centipede, Luoshiteng (Caulis Trachelospermi) 30 g, Danggui (Chinese Angelica) 30 g, Fangfeng (Radix Ledebouriellae) 10 g, and Honghua (Flos Carthami) 10 g.

Function: To warm meridians, release stagnation in collaterals, tone the blood, and expel wind pathogen.

Method of manipulation: A hot decoction of these herbs is used to steam and then wash both hands for 20-30 minutes, two to three times a day.

33. Tetany

This is a disease with convulsion of the limbs, stiffness of neck and back, and opisthotonos.

Diseases with convulsion of the limbs in modern medicine can be treated by the following methods.

Applications of hand therapy:

1) Acupuncture therapy:

(1) At regular and extra acupoints:

Location: Quchi (LI 11), Neiguan (PC 6), Houxi (SI 3) and Hegu (LI 4). Bleeding therapy may be applied at Shixuan (EX-UE 11).

Method of manipulation: The needles are inserted and retained for 20 minutes.

(2) At special acupoints beside the second metacarpal bone:

Location: Head acupoint, neck acupoint, upper limb acupoint, and leg acupoint.

Method of manipulation: The needles are inserted for 1.6 cm and retained for 15 minutes.

34. Headache

This is a common symptom that may occur alone or in conjunction with many acute and chronic diseases. In this section, only the treatment of headache with medical diseases is discussed.

Headache with epidemic and infectious diseases with fever, hypertension, intracranial diseases, neurasthenia, and migraine in modern medicine can be treated by the following methods.

Applications of hand therapy:

1) Massage therapy:

Location: Yuji (LU 10), Hegu (LI 4), Yangxi (LI 5), Shaoze (SI 1), Qiangu (SI 2), Houxi (SI 3), head reflective point (forehead, parietal head, temporal head and occipital head), brain area, head acupoint beside the second metacarpal bone, Guanchong (TE 1) and kidney area.

Method of manipulation: Both hands are rubbed to produce a hot sensation. Digit-pressing and kneading maneuvers applied at head area and kidney area; kneading and pressing maneuvers at Hegu (LI 4), Yangxi (LI 5), Shaoze (SI 1), Qiangu (SI 2), Houxi (SI 3), various head reflective points, brain area, Guanchong (TE 1) and head acupoint beside the second metacarpal bone 30-50 times. The acupoints, points, and areas may be selected according to the location of the headache.

2) Acupuncture therapy:

(1) At regular and extra acupoints:

Location: Hegu (LI 4) for frontal headache; Houxi (SI 3) for occipital headache; and Zhongdu (TE 3) for temporal headache.

Method of manipulation: The needles are retained for 30 minutes after strong needling stimulation.

(2) At reflective points:

Location: Forehead point for frontal headache; occipital head point for occipital headache; temporal head point for temporal headache; and parietal head point for parietal headache.

Method of manipulation: The needles are inserted for 1.6 cm and retained for five minutes after strong needling stimulation.

(3) At reflective areas:

Location: Head areas corresponding to the location of headache in dorsal and palmar reflective areas.

Method of manipulation: The needles are inserted and removed right after twisting, lifting, and thrusting stimulation.

(4) At special acupoint beside the second metacarpal bone:

Location: Head acupoint.

Method of manipulation: The needle is inserted for 1.6 cm and retained for 30 minutes.

3) Hand bath:

Recipe: Chuanxiong (Lovage) 40 g, Baizhi (Chinese Angelica) 10 g, Juhua (Chrysanthemum) 15 g, Baijiezi (white mustard seed) 10 g, Xixin (Herba Asari) 3 g, Shigao (Gypsum Fibrosum) 50 g, and scorpion 10 g.

Function: To disperse wind pathogen, clear heat pathogen, and stop pain.

Method of manipulation: A hot decoction is used to steam and then wash both hands for 20 minutes, twice a day.

4) Hand *qigong*: Kongjin exercise.

The hand is prone with the palm facing medially and the fingers relaxed and extended. The thumb is flexed twice and then resumes its starting posture; the little finger is flexed once and then resumes its original posture; and then the thumb is flexed once and resumes the original ladder pattern. The exercise is repeated 11 times and ended after a pole-standing exercise in riding posture for five minutes.

5) Herb-holding therapy:

Herbs: Qianghuo (Radix Notopterygii) 9 g, Duhuo (Radix Angelicae Tuhuo) 9 g, Chuanxiong (Lovage) 9 g, Xixin (Herba Asari) 6 g, and Fuzi (Aconite) 4 g.

Method of manipulation: A powder of the above herbs is mixed with a paste of green onion stalks and held in palms until some sweating is induced, twice a day.

35. Febrile diseases

The febrile diseases mentioned in this paragraph include chronic diseases with fever caused by dysfunction of the internal organs and deficiency of *qi*, blood, *yin* and *yang*.

Low fever, tumors, hematological diseases, diseases of connective tissues, tuberculosis, chronic infectious diseases, endocranial diseases, and diseases with fever of unknown origin in modern medicine can be treated by the following methods.

Applications of hand therapy:

Acupuncture therapy:

At regular and extra acupoints:

Location: Quchi (LI 11), Hegu (LI 4), Laogong (PC 8) and Yuji (LU 10) acupoints.

Method of manipulation: The needles are inserted and retained for 30 minutes after mild needling stimulation.

36. Malaria

Malaria is a disease with chills, high fever, headache and profuse sweating, usually occurring in summer and autumn.

Malaria and diseases with chills and high fever similar to malaria can be treated by the following methods.

Applications of hand therapy:

Acupuncture therapy:

At regular and extra acupoints:

Location: Houxi (SI 3), Jianshi (PC 5) and Quchi (LI 11) acupoints.

Method of manipulation: The needles are inserted two to three hours before the onset of chills and high fever and retained for 40 minutes.

37. Heat stroke

This is an acute disease with sudden onset of high fever, profuse sweating, mental confusion, sleepiness and sometimes convulsions due to the attack of summer-heat pathogen when working under a scorching sun or in a very hot environment. It is same as heat apoplexy in modern medicine and can be treated by the following methods.

Applications of hand therapy:

Acupuncture therapy:

(1) At regular and extra acupoints:

Location: Twelve *Jing* points or Shixuan (EX-UE 11), Quchi (LI 11) and Hegu (LI 4) acupoints.

Method of manipulation: Bleeding therapy is applied at 12 *Jing* points and Shixuan and routine acupuncture with strong needling stimulation is applied at Quchi and Hegu acupoints.

(2) At special acupoints beside the second metacarpal bone:

Location: Head acupoint and neck acupoint.

Method of manipulation: Bleeding therapy.

II. Dermatological and Surgical Conditions

1. Stiff neck

Stiff neck is most common in patients over 20 years of age and usually occurs in spring and autumn. It is often caused by an increase of local muscular tension or static injury to local tissues after sleeping in an improper posture or on an inadequate pillow. It can also be caused by attack of wind and cold pathogen in winter or even in summer to produce stagnation of *qi* and blood, blockage of meridians, functional disturbance, and pain and stiffness of the neck. The symptoms are pain in the neck and shoulder after sleeping, deviation of head to one side and limited neck movement. If the patient want to look backward, he must turn his body together with the head at the same time.

Cervical fascitis is the same disease and can be treated by the following methods.

Applications of hand therapy:

Acupuncture therapy:

(1) At regular and extra acupoints:

Location: Waiguan (TE 5), Houxi (SI 3), Zhongdu (TE 3) or pierced from Yemen (TE 2) to Zhongdu (TE 3).

Method of manipulation: The strong needling stimulation is applied and accompanied by local exercise.

(2) At reflective point.

Location: Neck reflective point.

Method of manipulation: The needle is inserted for 1.6 cm for application of strong needling stimulation and accompanied by local exercise.

(3) At special acupoint beside the second metacarpal bone.

Location: Neck acupoint beside the second metacarpal bone.

Method of manipulation: The needle is inserted for 1.6 cm and retained for 15 minutes.

2. Furuncle

This is a pyogenic disease of the skin with multiple lesions and repeated relapses. The infection may last for a long time with new lesions repeatedly appearing after the old lesions have healed. In traditional Chinese medicine, the furuncles occurring along the posterior hairline are called *Faji Chuang* (hairline sores) and those over the buttocks are called *Zuoban Chuang* (ischial sores). This disease is most common in young people.

The pyogenic infection of single hair follicles and sweat glands in modern medicine is the same disease and can be treated by the following methods.

Applications of hand therapy:

1) Acupuncture therapy:

(1) At regular and extra acupoints:

Location: Ximen (PC 4), Quchi (LI 11), Hegu (LI 4) and Zhoujian (EX-UE 1) acupoints.

Method of manipulation: The strong needling stimulation is applied.

(2) At reflective areas:

Location: Areas corresponding to the location of furuncles in dorsal and palmar reflective areas.

Method of manipulation: The regular needles are used for routine acupuncture and the three-edged needle is used for bleeding therapy.

2) Hand bath:

Recipe: Lianqiao (Fructus Forsythia) 15 g, Jinyinhua (Flos Lonicerae) 20 g, Pugongying (Herba Taraxaci) 15 g, Huangbo (Cortex Phellodendri) 15 g, Kushen (Shrub of Sophora) 15 g, Niuxi (Radix Achyranthis Bidentatae) 15 g, and Chuanjiao (Pericarpium Zanthoxyli) 6 g.

Function: To clear heat pathogen and dispel toxic pathogen.

Method of manipulation: A hot decoction of the above herbs is used to steam and wash both hands for 20-30 minutes, twice a day.

3. Tuberculosis of cervical lymph nodes

This is a chronic infectious disease, most common in children and youths. The onset of the disease is insidious, and at the beginning a painless and beanlike nodule covered with normal skin appears. Then it gradually grows in size with more lesions appearing and the skin turns dark red after suppuration of the lesions. The suppurative lesions may rupture and discharge thin pus with flocculent material. Some ruptured lesions may heal, while other new lesions may rupture.

Tuberculosis of the cervical lymph nodes may be treated by the following methods.

Applications of hand therapy:

1) Acupuncture therapy:

(1) At regular and extra acupoints:

Location: Tianjing (TE 10), Zhoujian (EX-UE 1) and Quchi (LI 11) acupoints.

Method of manipulation: Routine acupuncture and bleeding therapy may be applied.

(2) At reflective areas:

Location: Areas according to the correspondent location of lesions in dorsal and palmar reflective areas.

Method of manipulation: Routine acupuncture and bleeding therapy may be applied.

4. Acute mastitis

This is an acute pyogenic infection of the breasts in breast-feeding women, usually occurring three to four months after childbirth and most common in first pregnancies.

Acute mastitis in modern medicine can be treated by the following methods.

1) Massage therapy:

Location: Chest, liver, breast, and lymph node areas, interosseous spaces on palm, and tender spots.

Method of manipulation: Pressing and kneading maneuvers applied to the chest, liver, breast, and lymph node areas; pushing and pressing interosseous spaces on palm; and digit-pressing maneuver at tender spots. This manipulation may be repeatedly applied.

2) Acupuncture therapy:

(1) At regular and extra acupoints:

Location: Neiguan (PC 6), Hegu (LI 4) and Quchi (LI 11).

Method of manipulation: The strong stimulation is applied and the needles are retained for 30 minutes.

(2) At reflective point.

Location: Chest reflective point.

Method of manipulation: The needle is inserted for 1.6 cm and retained for five minutes.

(3) At reflective areas:

Location: Breast area in palmar reflective areas and radial and ulnar reverse palmar reflective areas.

Method of manipulation: Routine acupuncture and bleeding therapy may be applied.

3) Hand bath:

Recipe: Liujinu (Herba Artemisiae Anomalae) 30 g, Pugongying (Herba Taraxaci) 60 g, Zihuadiding (Radix et Herba Violae) 30 g, Honghua (Flos Carthami) 10 g, and Ruxiang (Frankincence) 10 g.

Function: To clear heat pathogen, relieve intoxication, release blood stasis, and stop pain.

Method of manipulation: The herbs are wrapped in gauze and boiled in water to prepare a hot decoction for application of steaming and washing therapy to both hands and affected breast for 30 minutes, two to three times a day. This therapy can produce a good effect at the early stages of acute mastitis.

5. Herpes zoster

This is an acute skin disease with burning pain. The skin lesions are the erythema and clusters of vesicles arranged in tapelike around the trunk of the body.

Applications of hand therapy:

Acupuncture therapy:

(1) At regular and extra acupoints:

Location: According to the location of lesions. For example, Quchi (LI 11) and Hegu (LI 4) for lesions on the face; and Zhigou (TE 6), Waiguan (TE 5) and Houxi (SI 3) for lesions on the waist.

Method of manipulation: After strong stimulation, the needles are retained for 30 minutes.

(2) At reflective areas:

Location: Areas corresponding to the location of lesion in dorsal and palmar reflective areas.

Method of manipulation: Routine acupuncture and bleeding therapy can be applied.

6. Eczema

This is a chronic, recurring, and irritating skin disease. The multiform skin lesions are symmetrically distributed, with erosion and oozing.

Acute and chronic allergic skin diseases can be treated by the following methods.

Applications of hand therapy:

1) Massage therapy:

Location: Tender spots, kidney, stomach, intestine, spleen, and lung areas.

Method of manipulation: Pressing and kneading maneuvers are applied at above areas and points.

2) Acupuncture therapy:

(1) At regular and extra acupoints:

Location: Quchi (LI 11), Hegu (LI 4) and Zhoujian (EX-UE 1) acupoints.

Method of manipulation: The strong stimulation is applied.

(2) At special acupoints beside the second metacarpal bone:

Location: According to the location of the lesion. For example, the upper limb acupoint is used for lesions on upper limbs; and the head acupoint is used for lesions of the head.

Method of manipulation: Bleeding therapy is applied.

3) Hand bath:

Recipe: Kushen (Radix Sophorae) 30 g, Baixianpi (Cortex Dictamni Radicis) 30 g, Difuzi (Fructus Kochiae) 30 g, Tufuling (Rhizoma Smilacis Glabrae) 30 g, Shechuangzi (Fructus Cnidii) 30 g, Chantui (Periostracum Cicadae) 15 g, Huangqing (Radix Scutellariae) 15 g, Pugongying (Herba Taraxaci) 30 g, and Baibu (Radix Stemonae) 20 g.

Function: To clear heat pathogen, relieve toxicity, resolve dampness, and stop itching.

Method of manipulation: The herbs are wrapped in gauze and boiled in water for steaming and washing both hands and skin lesions for 30 minutes, twice a day.

7. Urticaria

This is a skin disease with pink or pale papules appearing on the skin and then disappearing from time to time.

Urticaria in modern medicine can be treated by the following methods.

Applications of hand therapy:

1) Massage therapy:

Location: Lung, liver, stomach, intestine areas, and lung reflective point.

Method of manipulation: Both hands are rubbed to produce

a hot sensation. Digit-pressing maneuver applied at lung, liver, stomach, and intestine areas 50 times at each area.

2) Acupuncture therapy:

At regular and extra acupoints:

Location: Quchi (LI 11), Hegu (LI 4) and Houxi (SI 3) acupoints.

Method of manipulation: The needles are inserted and retained for 30 minutes.

3) Hand bath:

Recipe: Jingjie (Herba Schizonepetae) 15 g, Fangfeng (Radix Ledebouriellae) 15 g, Shigao (Gypsum Fibrosum) 30 g, Zhimu (Rhizoma Anemarrhenae) 10 g, Baixianpi (Cortex Dictamni Radicis) 20 g, Kushen (Radix Sophorae) 30 g, Difuzi (Fructus Kochiae) 20 g, Dafengzi (Semen Hydnocapi) 15 g, Gancao (Licorice) 10 g, and Chantui (Periostracum Cicadae) 10 g.

Function: To resolve dampness, clear heat pathogen, expel wind pathogen, and stop itching.

Method of manipulation: These herbs are wrapped in gauze and boiled in an adequate amount of water to prepare a hot decoction for steaming and then washing both hands for 30 minutes. When the decoction cools, the boiled water may be added for further steaming and washing manipulation, and the hand bath may be applied two to three times a day.

8. Neurodermatitis

In traditional Chinese medicine this is called *niupi* (ox skin) *xuan*, because the skin lesion is tough and thick like the skin of an ox. It is also called *sheling* (around the neck) *chuang*, because it usually occurs in the neck and nape region.

Neurodermatitis in modern medicine can be treated by the following methods.

Applications of hand therapy:

1) Massage therapy:

Location: Head, neck, spine, lymph and immunity, and lung areas, and heart and chest region.

Method of manipulation: The digit-pressing maneuver is applied to all of these areas and regions.

2) Acupuncture therapy:

(1) At regular and extra acupoints:

Location: Quchi (LI 11), Hegu (LI 4) and Houxi (SI 3) acupoints.

Method of manipulation: The needles are inserted and retained for 30 minutes.

(2) At special acupoints beside the second metacarpal bone:

Location: According to the location of the skin lesion. For example, the neck acupoint is used for lesion in the neck region.

3) Hand bath:

Recipe: Zaojiao (Fructus Gleditsiae) 30 g, Kushen (Radix Shrub) 15 g, Shechuangzi (Fructus Cnidii) 15 g, Tujinpi (Cortex Pseudolaricis) 15 g, Baibu (Radix Stemonae) 20 g, Dafengzi (Semen Hydnocapi) 15 g, and Lingxiaohuateng (Caulis Campsis) 30 g.

Function: To expel wind, resolve dampness, kill parasites and stop itching.

Method of manipulation: A hot decoction of these herbs is used to steam and wash both hands for 30 minutes, two to three times a day.

9. Tinea manuum

In traditional Chinese medicine this is called *ezhang* (goose claw) *feng*, because the skin lesion on hand is rough and scattered with fissures like the claw of a goose.

Tinea manuum in modern medicine can be treated by the following methods.

1) Acupuncture therapy:

(1) At regular and extra acupoints:

Location: Hegu (LI 4), Yuji (LU 10), Laogong (PC 8) and Quchi (LI 11) acupoints.

Method of manipulation: After medium stimulation, the needles are retained for 30 minutes, once a day for 10 days as a therapeutic course.

(2) At reflective points:

Location: Lung point, anti-itching point, and heart point.

Method of manipulation: Routine acupuncture is applied two to three times a day for seven days as a therapeutic course.

(3) At special acupoints beside the second metacarpal bone:
Location: Lung acupoint and tender spots.

Method of manipulation: The needles are inserted for 1.6 cm and retained for 15-30 minutes after strong stimulation, once a day for 10 days as a therapeutic course.

3) Hand bath:

Recipe: Dafengzi (Semen Hydnocapi) 15 g, Huajiao (Pericarpium Zanthoxyli) 9 g, Zaojia (Fructus Gleditsiae) 15 g, Tujinpi (Cortex Pseudolaricis) 15 g, Digupi (Cortex Lycii Radicis) 6 g, Baifan (Alumen) 12 g, Yeqiangweigen (Radix Rosae Multiflorae, wild) 30 g, and Huoxiang (Herba Agastachis) 15 g.

Function: To expel wind, resolve dampness, clear heat, and tone *yin*.

Method of manipulation: A hot decoction of these herbs is used to steam and wash both hands for 30 minutes, two to three times a day.

III. Gynecological Diseases

1. Dysmenorrhea

This is a disease in women characterized by lower abdominal pain before, during, or after the menstrual period. The pain may radiated to lumbar and sacral regions, and severe pain may cause fainting. It is also called menstrual abdominal pain.

Dysmenorrhea often occurs in patients with hypoplasia of the uterus, extreme anteversion or retroversion of uterus, narrowed cervical canal, menstrual discharge with flakes of endometrium, endometriosis, and pelvic inflammation.

Applications of hand therapy:

1) Massage therapy:

Location: Kidney, reproductive, and reproductive gland areas, thenar and hypothenar prominences, interosseous space between the fourth and fifth metacarpal bones, uterus reflective point, and cardiac palpitation point.

Method of manipulation: Both hands are rubbed to produce a hot sensation. Pushing and pressing thenar and hypothenar prominences; heavy pressing maneuver applied at kidney, reproductive, and reproductive gland areas; pinching and pressing maneuvers at interosseous space between fourth and fifth metacarpal bones; and heavy pinching maneuver at uterus and cardiac palpitation points.

2) Acupuncture therapy:

(1) At regular and extra acupoint:

Location: Hegu (LI 4) acupoint.

Method of manipulation: The needle is inserted for 3.3 cm to apply strong needling stimulation.

(2) At reflective points:

Location: Triple energizer point and waist point.

Method of manipulation: The needles are inserted for 1 cm to apply medium needling stimulation.

(3) At acupoint beside the second metacarpal bone:

Location: Lower abdomen acupoint.

Method of manipulation: The needle is inserted for 3.3 cm and retained for 20 minutes after twisting, lifting, and thrusting stimulation.

3) Hand bath:

Recipe: Shanzha (Fructus Crataegi) 30 g, Honghua (Flos Carthami) 10 g, Wulingzhi (Faeces Togopterorum) 15 g, Sumu (Lignum Sappan) 15 g, Yanhusuo (Rhizoma Corydalis) 15 g, Mike (Fructus Papaveris) 20 g, Xuejie (Sanguis Draconis) 20 g, and dried ginger 10 g.

Function: To promote blood circulation, release blood stasis, warm meridians, and stop pain.

Method of manipulation: A hot decoction of these herbs is used to steam and wash both hands for 20-30 minutes, two to three times a day.

2. Menstrual headache

This is a condition with headache before, during, or after the menstrual period due to blood deficiency, stagnant blood, and fire pathogen in the liver.

Premenstrual tension in modern medicine is same as this disease and can be treated by the following methods.

Applications of hand therapy:

1) Massage therapy:

Location: Reproductive, kidney, and head areas, uterus reflective point, Mingmen point, Hegu (LI 4), Shaoze (SI 1), Qiangu (SI 2), Houxi (SI 3), Yemen (TE 2) and various head reflective points.

Method of manipulation: Both hands are rubbed to produce a hot sensation. Pushing and grinding maneuvers applied at reproductive, kidney, and head areas; digit-pressing maneuver at uterus reflective point, Mingmen point, Hegu (LI 4), Shaoze (SI 1), Qiangu (SI 2), Houxi (SI 3), Yemen (TE 2) and various head reflective points.

2) Acupuncture therapy:

(1) At regular and extra acupoints:

Location: Hegu (LI 4) and Houxi (SI 3) acupoints.

Method of manipulation: The medium stimulation is applied and the needles are retained for 30 minutes.

(2) At reflective areas:

Location: Head area corresponding to the location of headache in dorsal and palmar reflective areas.

Method of manipulation: The needle is shallowly inserted and removed right after the twisting, lifting, and thrusting stimulation.

(3) At acupoints beside the second metacarpal bone:

Location: Head acupoint and liver acupoint.

Method of manipulation: The needles are inserted for 3.3 cm and retained for 20 minutes.

3) Hand bath:

Recipe: Chuanxiong (Rhizoma Ligustici) 30 g, Xiangfu (Rhizoma Cyperi) 20 g, Wuzhuyu (Evodia) 20 g, Huajiao (Pericarpium Zanthoxyli) 6 g, and fresh stalks of green onion 30 g.

Function: To disperse stagnation of liver *qi*, promote blood circulation, and stop pain.

Method of manipulation: A hot decoction of the above herbs is used to steam and wash both hands and head for 20 minutes, two to three times a day.

3. Amenorrhea

This is a condition in which menstruation has not begun in girls over 18 years of age, or with menstruation discontinued over three months in women having regular menstruation in the past.

Amenorrhea in modern medicine can be divided into primary and secondary types. The latter type is secondary to various diseases which should be properly administered to specific treatment. The cessation of menstruation in pregnant and breast-feeding women is a normal phenomenon and not included in pathological amenorrhea. Amenorrhea in patients with congenital absence of uterus, ovaries, or vagina and imperforate hymen is due to special organic lesions and cannot be cured by hand therapy.

Applications of hand therapy:

1) Massage therapy:

Location: Reproductive area, kidney area, wrist and uterus reflective points, and Hegu (LI 4).

Method of manipulation: Both hands are rubbed to produce a hot sensation. Rubbing maneuver applied to wrists; grinding and pushing maneuvers at reproductive area and kidney area; and digit-pressing and kneading maneuvers at uterus point and Hegu (LI 4).

2) Acupuncture therapy:

(1) At regular and extra acupoints:

Location: Hegu (LI 4) and Houxi (SI 3) acupoints.

Method of manipulation: The strong stimulation is applied and the needles are retained for 30 minutes.

(2) At reflective points:

Location: Kidney point, spine point, and liver point.

Method of manipulation: The needles are inserted for 1.3 cm and retained for five minutes after medium stimulation.

(3) At acupoint beside the second metacarpal bone:

Location: Lower abdomen acupoint.

Method of manipulation: The needle is inserted for 1.6-3.3 cm and retained for 20 minutes.

4. Postpartum bleeding shock

After delivery, the mother may suddenly develop dizziness, blurred vision, difficulty sitting up, chest distress, nausea, vomiting, shortness of breath with accumulation of phlegm, restlessness, or and even trismus, loss of consciousness, and coma.

Applications of hand therapy:

1) Massage therapy:

Location: Heart, stomach, kidney, reproductive and reproductive gland areas, and brain, head and stomach reflective points.

Method of manipulation: Both hands are rubbed to produce a hot sensation. Rubbing maneuver applied to palm root; digit-pressing and kneading heart, stomach, kidney and reproductive areas and reproductive gland area; continuous digit-pressing and kneading brain, head and stomach reflective point.

2) Acupuncture therapy:

(1) At regular and extra acupoints:

Location: Neiguan (PC 6), Hegu (LI 4), Kongzui (LU 6) and Yinxi (HT 6) acupoints.

Method of manipulation: The weak stimulation is applied and the needles are retained for 15 minutes.

(2) At reflective points:

Location: Heart, spleen, and kidney points.

Method of manipulation: The needles are shallowly inserted and retained for five minutes.

(3) At special acupoints beside the second metacarpal bone:

Location: Head acupoint, liver acupoint and lung and heart acupoint.

Method of manipulation: The needles are inserted for 1.6 cm

and retained for 15 minutes after weak stimulation.

3) Hand bath:

Recipe: Danggui (Chinese Angelica) 60 g, Dangshen (Radix Codonopsis Pilosulae) 20 g, Fuling (Poria) 20 g, Juhua (Chrysanthemum) 10 g, and Chishao (Radix Paeoniae Rubra) 10 g.

Function: To tone *qi* and blood and improve vision.

Method of manipulation: A hot decoction of the above herbs is used to steam and wash both hands for 30 minutes, two to three times a day.

4) Hand *qigong*: Kongjin exercise.

The hand is prone with the palm facing downward and the fingers relaxed and extended. The thumb and little finger are flexed at the same time seven times (Fig. 49); and the middle and little fingers are flexed at the same time six times (Fig. 50). The hand should be returned to the ladder pattern after each repetition and the exercise is ended after a pole-standing exercise in the riding posture for five minutes.

5. Postpartum convulsions

This is a condition in new mothers with convulsions of the limbs, stiffness of neck and back, trismus, and opisthotonos.

Postpartum convulsions and postpartum tetanus can be treated by the following methods.

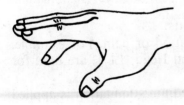

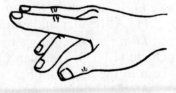

Fig. 49   Fig. 50

Applications of hand therapy:

1) Acupuncture therapy:

(1) At regular and extra acupoints:

Location: Quchi (LI 11), Hegu (LI 4), Houxi (SI 3) and Neiguan (PC 6) acupoints.

Method of manipulation: The medium stimulation is applied and the needles are retained for 20 minutes.

(2) At special acupoints beside the second metacarpal bone:

Location: Upper limb acupoint, leg acupoint, and liver acupoint.

Method of manipulation: The needles are inserted for 1.6 cm and retained for 20 minutes.

2) Hand bath:

Recipe: Danggui (Chinese Angelica) 100 g, Tianma (Rhizoma Gastrodiae) 10 g, scorpion 10 g, silkworm 15 g, centipede 2 pieces, and Nanxing (Rhizoma Arisaematis) 10 g.

Function: To promote blood circulation, tone the blood and control convulsions due to disturbance of internal wind pathogen.

Method of manipulation: A hot decoction of these herbs is used to steam and wash both hands for 30 minutes, twice a day.

6. Body pain after childbirth

Body pain in women after childbirth with soreness, numbness, and heaviness of body, also called postpartum pain, caused by wind pathogen, can be treated by the following methods.

Applications of hand therapy:

1) Acupuncture therapy:

(1) At regular and extra acupoints:

Location: According to the location of pain. For example, Quchi (LI 11), Waiguan (TE 5) and Hegu (LI 4) are used for pain in the upper limbs.

Method of manipulation: The medium stimulation is applied and the needles are retained for 20 minutes.

(2) At reflective areas:

Location: According to the location of pain, the areas corresponding to the location of pain in the dorsal reflective areas and ulnar or radial reverse dorsal reflective areas.

Method of manipulation: The needles are shallowly inserted and not retained after needling stimulation.

(3) At special acupoints beside the second metacarpal bone:

Location: According to the location of pain, the upper limb acupoint, waist acupoint, or leg acupoint can be selected.

Method of manipulation: The needles are inserted for 1.6 cm and retained for 20 minutes after medium needling stimulation.

2) Hand bath:

Recipe: Qingfengteng (Caulis Sinomenii) 30 g, Haifengteng (Caulis Piperis Dadsurae) 30 g, Luoshiteng (Caulis Trachelospermi) 30 g, Weilingxian (Chinese Clematis) 15 g, Qinjiao (Radix Gentianae Macrophyllae) 20 g, Renseng (Radix Ginseng) 10 g, Danggui (Chinese Angelica) 60 g, Chuanwu (Radix Aconiti) 10 g and Caowu (Jack-in-the-Pulpit) 10 g.

Function: To tone *qi* and blood, expel wind and dampness pathogens, warm meridians, and stop pain.

Method of manipulation: A hot decoction of these herbs is used to steam and wash both hands for 30 minutes, twice a day.

7. Oligogalactia

After childbirth, a lessening or complete lack of milk in new mothers can be treated by the following methods.

Applications of hand therapy:

1) Massage therapy:

Location: Palm, palm root, head, kidney, and liver areas, Shaoze (SI 1) and Qiangu (SI 2) acupoints.

Method of manipulation: Both hands are rubbed to produce a hot sensation. Rubbing palm, kneading and pressing palm root, pushing and rubbing maneuvers applied to head, kidney, and liver areas; and digit-pressing, kneading, twisting, and rubbing maneuvers at Shaoze (SI 1) and Qiangu (SI 2) acupoints.

2) Acupuncture therapy:

(1) At regular and extra acupoints:

Location: Neiguan (PC 6), Hegu (LI 4) and Shaoze (SI 1) acupoints.

Method of manipulation: Bleeding therapy is applied at Shaoze; and routine acupuncture is applied at other acupoints for 30 minutes.

(2) At reflective points:

Location: Chest point and liver point.

Method of manipulation: The needles are inserted for 1 cm and retained for five minutes.

(3) At special acupoints beside the second metacarpal bone:

Location: Lung and heart acupoint, liver acupoint, and stomach acupoint.

Method of manipulation: The needles are inserted for 1.6 cm and retained for 20 minutes.

3) Hand bath:

Recipe: Loulu (Radix Phapontici) 20 g, Tianhuafen (Radix Trichosanthis) 30 g, Baizhi (Chinese Angelica) 20 g, Danggui (Chinese Angelica) 60 g, Xiangfu (Rhizoma Cyperi) 15 g, Lulutong (Fructus Liquidambaris) 20 g, and half a pig's foot.

Function: To tone the blood, release stagnation in meridians, and promote the discharge of milk.

Method of manipulation: These herbs are boiled for 60 minutes and the hot decoction is used to steam and wash both hands for 20-30 minutes, three times a day for seven days.

8. Infertility in women

This is a condition of women unable to become pregnant after living together with a healthy husband with no reproductive abnormalities for more than two years and without using contraception.

Applications of hand therapy:

1) Massage therapy:

Location: Kidney, reproductive, reproductive gland areas, and wrist reflective joint.

Method of manipulation: Both hands are rubbed to produce a hot sensation. Digit-pressing maneuver applied at kidney area, reproductive area, and reproductive gland area; rubbing wrist joint; pushing and kneading maneuvers at thenar and hypothenar regions; and pinching and twisting the little fingers.

2) Acupuncture therapy:

(1) At reflective points:

Location: Spleen point, kidney point, and liver point.

Method of manipulation: The needles are inserted for 1.3 cm and retained for five minutes after medium needling stimulation.

(2) At reflective areas:

Location: Lower abdomen area in palmar reflective areas and radial or ulnar reverse palmar reflective areas.

Method of manipulation: The needles are shallowly inserted and not retained.

(3) At special acupoints beside the second metacarpal bone:

Location: Liver acupoint, kidney acupoint and lower abdomen acupoint.

Method of manipulation: The needles are inserted for 2.6 cm and retained for 30 minutes.

9. Abdominal mass

In traditional Chinese medicine, masses in the lower abdomen in women can be divided into two types: *Zheng* masses which are hard, fixed, cause pain in a specific location, and form due to a disturbance of blood; and *Jia* masses which are movable, cause general pain, and form due to the disturbance of *qi*. These two types of masses are closely related and cannot be absolutely distinguished one from the other.

Ovarian cysts, adnexitis, and pelvic inflammation are similar to this disease and can be treated by the following methods.

Applications of hand therapy:

1) Acupuncture therapy:

(1) At regular and extra acupoints:

Location: Neiguan (PC 6), Hegu (LI 4) and Quchi (LI 11) acupoints.

Method of manipulation: The needles are retained for 20

minutes after strong needling stimulation.

(2) At special acupoint beside the second metacarpal bone:

Location: Lower abdomen acupoint.

Method of manipulation: The needle is inserted for 3.3 cm and retained for 30 minutes after strong stimulation.

IV. Pediatric Diseases

1. Convulsions

This is a common symptom in children with convulsions and mental confusion. The progression of this disease is rapid and may be considered life-threatening. The incidence is highest among young children. In traditional Chinese medicine, it is divided into the acute type with *yang* and excessive nature called acute convulsion; and the chronic type with *yin* and deficient nature called chronic convulsion.

Convulsions in children and convulsions due to deficiency of calcium and other causes in modern medicine can be treated by the following methods.

Applications of hand therapy:

Acupuncture therapy:

(1) At regular and extra acupoints:

Location: Twelve *Jing* acupoints, Shixuan (EX-UE 11), Neiguan (PC 6) and Hegu (LI 4) acupoints.

Method of manipulation: Bleeding therapy is applied at 12 *Jing* acupoints and Shixuan (EX-UE 11) and the routine acupuncture is applied to other acupoints with the needles not retained.

(2) At special acupoints beside the second metacarpal bone:

Location: Head acupoint, upper limb acupoint, and leg acupoint.

Method of manipulation: The needles are inserted for 1.6 cm and retained for five minutes after twisting, lifting, and thrusting stimulation.

2. Anorexia

This is a disease in children characterized by poor appetite and even a refusal to eat over a long period of time.

Applications of hand therapy:

Acupuncture therapy:

(1) At regular and extra acupoints:

Location: Shousanli (LI 10), Hegu (LI 4) and Sifeng (EX-UE 10) acupoints.

Method of manipulation: Bleeding therapy is applied at Sifeng acupoints and routine acupuncture is applied at other acupoints.

(2) At reflective points:

Location: Stomach and intestine point and spleen point.

Method of manipulation: The needles are inserted for 1 cm, but not retained.

(3) At special acupoint beside the second metacarpal bone:

Location: Stomach acupoint.

Method of manipulation: The needle is inserted for 1.6 cm, but not retained.

3. Stagnation of food

The symptoms of this condition are poor appetite, indigestion, abdominal distension, and irregular bowel movement.

Indigestion and malnutrition in children in modern medicine are same as food stagnation and can be treated by the following methods.

Applications of hand therapy:

Acupuncture therapy:

(1) At regular and extra acupoints:

Location: Sifeng (EX-UE 10) and Hegu (LI 4) acupoints.

Method of manipulation: Bleeding therapy is applied at Sifeng (EX-UE 10) acupoints to squeeze out blood and serum, and routine acupuncture is applied at Hegu (LI 4) with needle not retained.

(2) At special acupoint beside the second metacarpal bone:

Location: Stomach acupoint.

Method of manipulation: The needle is inserted for 1.6 cm, but not retained.

4. Indigestive malnutrition

This is a common chronic disease of children with general weakness and pathological leanness, sallow complexion, and dry hair due to improper feeding. It may be caused by many different diseases.

Malnutrition in children, nutritional anemia, and chronic indigestion in modern medicine can be treated by the following methods.

Applications of hand therapy:

1) Acupuncture therapy:

(1) At regular and extra acupoint:

Location: Sifeng (EX-UE 10) acupoints.

Method of manipulation: Bleeding therapy is applied at Sifeng (EX-UE 10) acupoints to squeeze out blood and serum.

(2) At special acupoints beside the second metacarpal bone:

Location: Stomach and intestine acupoint, spleen acupoint, and triple energizer acupoint.

Method of manipulation: The needles are shallowly inserted, but not retained.

2) Herb-holding therapy:

Herbs: Dahuang (Rhubarb) 9 g, Qianniuzi (Semen Pharbitidis) 12 g, and Laifuzi (Radish Seed) 10 g.

Method of manipulation: The herbs are ground to powder and wrapped in gauze for holding in palms by older children or fixed to palms by a bandage for young babies.

5. Poliomyelitis

In the preparalytic stage, the child may suffer from fever, cough, red throat, and general muscular pain. This is often accompanied by vomiting and diarrhea and flaccid muscles and weak limbs. In the later stages, the significant symptoms are muscular atrophy and bone deformity.

Applications of hand therapy:

Acupuncture therapy:

(1) At regular and extra acupoints:

Location: According to the involved limbs, Quchi (LI 11),

Waiguan (TE 5) and Hegu (LI 4) for paralysis of upper limb; and Quchi and Houxi (SI 3) acupoints for paralysis of lower limb. The paralytic limbs should be either actively or passively moved during application of acupuncture.

Method of manipulation: The medium stimulation is applied and the needles are not retained.

(2) At special acupoints beside the second metacarpal bone:

Location: According to the involved limbs, upper limb acupoint is used for paralysis of upper limb, and leg acupoint and waist acupoint are used for paralysis of lower limb.

6. Retardation of development

This condition includes the retardation of standing, walking, and speaking, and retarded growth of hair and teeth.

Maldevelopment of children in modern medicine can be treated by the following methods.

Applications of hand therapy:

Acupuncture therapy:

(1) At regular and extra acupoints:

Location: Shousanli (LI 10), Hegu (LI 4) and Sifeng (EX-UE 10) acupoints.

Method of manipulation: Bleeding therapy is applied at Sifeng (EX-UE 10); and routine acupuncture is applied at Shousanli (LI 10) and Hegu (LI 4) acupoints with weak stimulation, and needles not retained.

(2) At special acupoints beside the second metacarpal bone:

Location: Heart, stomach, and kidney acupoints.

Method of manipulation: The needles are inserted for 1.6 cm, but not retained.

7. General weakness

This condition includes weakness of neck, mouth, arms, legs, and muscles.

Rickets, congenital hydrocephalus, and congenital maldevelopment in modern medicine are similar to this condition and can be treated by the methods mentioned for retardation of development.

8. Scleroderma in newborns

Newborns with this disease may have hardness of neck, mouth, hands, feet and muscles.

Newborn scleroderma in modern medicine can be treated by the following methods.

Applications of hand therapy:

Acupuncture therapy:

(1) At regular and extra acupoints:

Location: Quchi (LI 11), Neiguan (PC 6), Houxi (SI 3) and Hegu (LI 4) acupoints.

Method of manipulation: Moxibustion with moxa roll can be applied at above acupoints.

(2) At special acupoints beside the second metacarpal bone:

Location: Upper limb, leg, spleen, and kidney acupoints.

Method of manipulation: The needles are inserted for 1.6 cm and a short piece of moxa roll is attached to the handle of needle for application of moxibustion; the gentle moxibustion or pecking moxibustion with moxa roll is applied at above special acupoints.

V. Diseases of the Eye, Ear, Nose, and Oral Cavity

1. Tinnitus and deafness

Patients with tinnitus may have auditory hallucinations. Deafness is a hearing impairment of varying severity—from a slight reduction to a complete loss of hearing.

Perceptive and mixed deafness in modern medicine can be treated by the following methods.

Applications of hand therapy:

1) Massage therapy:

Location: Throat, ear, lung, stomach, and intestinal areas, head reflective point, Shangyang (LI 1), Hegu (LI 4), Yangxi (LI 5), Qiangu (SI 2), Houxi (SI 3), Shanghouxi (EX acupoint), Wangu (SI 4), Yanggu (SI 5), Zhongdu (TE 3), and Yangchi (TE 4) acupoints.

Method of manipulation: Digit-pressing maneuver applied at throat, ear, lung, stomach, and intestinal areas; twisting and pinching middle and ring fingers; pinching and kneading maneuvers applied at Shangyang (LI 1), Hegu (LI 4), Yangxi (LI 5), Qiangu (SI 2), Houxi (SI 3), Shanghouxi (EX acupoint), Wangu (SI 4), Yanggu (SI 5), Zhongdu (TE 3), and Yangchi (TE 4) acupoints; and digit-pressing and pinching maneuvers at head reflective point.

2) Acupuncture therapy:

(1) At regular and extra acupoints:

Location: Yemen (TE 2), Zhongdu (TE 3) and Waiguan (TE 5) acupoints.

Method of manipulation: The medium stimulation is applied and the needles are retained for 30 minutes.

(2) At reflective points:

Location: Temporal head point and kidney point.

Method of manipulation: The needles are inserted for 1.6 cm and retained for 15 minutes.

(3) At special acupoints beside the second metacarpal bone:

Location: Head acupoint and kidney acupoint.

Method of manipulation: The needles are inserted for 1.6 cm and retained for 20 minutes after medium needling stimulation.

2. Nasal obstruction

Nasal obstruction may be a chronic condition with repeated relapses. The size and severity of obstruction may change from time to time, and in severe cases the olfactory sense may be completely lost.

Chronic simple rhinitis and chronic hypertrophic rhinitis in modern medicine are similar to this disease and can be treated by the following methods.

Applications of hand therapy:

1) Massage therapy:

Location: Midline of palm, nose, throat, lung, and lymph areas, stomach and intestine reflective point, and head acupoint.

Method of manipulation: Pushing midline of palm; digit-pressing and kneading maneuvers applied at nose, throat, lung, and lymph areas; and pinching maneuver at stomach and intestine point and head acupoint.

2) Acupuncture therapy:

(1) At regular and extra acupoints:

Location: Shaoshang (LU 10) and Hegu (LI 4) acupoints.

Method of manipulation: Bleeding therapy is applied at Shaoshang; the needle is inserted at Hegu for 3.3 cm and retained for 30 minutes after strong needling stimulation.

(2) At special acupoints beside the second metacarpal bone:

Location: Head acupoint and liver acupoint.

Method of manipulation: The needles are inserted for 1.6 cm and retained for 20 minutes.

3. Atrophic rhinitis

This is a disease of the nose with dryness and foul smell in the nose, nasal obstruction, atrophy of nasal mucosa, and dilatation of nasal cavity.

Atrophic rhinitis in modern medicine can be treated by the methods mentioned for nasal obstruction.

4. Toothache

Toothache is a symptom of various diseases of the teeth and periodontal structures.

Applications of hand therapy:

1) Massage therapy:

Location: Toothache point, common cold point, Shangyang (LI 1), Hegu (LI 4), Erjian (LI 2), Sanjian (LI 3), Yangxi (LI 5), Houxi (SI 3), Shanghegu (EX point), and kidney area.

Method of manipulation: Pinching, digit-pressing and kneading maneuvers applied at toothache point, common cold point, Hegu (LI 4), Shangyang (LI 1), Erjian (LI 2), Sanjian (LI 3), Yangxi (LI 5), Houxi (SI 3) and Shanghegu (EX point) acupoints. A toothpick may be used to stimulate kidney point to reduce the pain in patients with an acute toothache attack.

2) Acupuncture therapy:

(1) At regular and extra acupoints:

Location: Shangyang (LI 1) and Hegu (LI 4) acupoints.

Method of manipulation: Bleeding therapy is applied at Shangyang (LI 1); and the needle is inserted at Hegu (LI 4) for application of strong needling stimulation and retained for 30 minutes.

(2) At reflective point:

Location: Toothache point.

Method of manipulation: The needle is inserted for 1 cm and retained for five minutes after strong stimulation.

3) Hand bath:

Recipe: Baizhi (Chinese Angelica) 15 g, Bibo (Fructus Piperis Longi) 20 g, Gaoliangjiang (Rhizoma Alliniae Officinarum) 20 g, Yanhusuo (Rhizoma Corydalis) 20 g, and Mike (Fructus Papaveris) 20 g.

Function: To warm meridians and stop pain.

Method of manipulation: A hot decoction is used to steam and wash both hands for 20-30 minutes, two to three times a day.

5. Acute laryngitis

This is an acute condition with hoarse voice and dysphonia.

Acute laryngitis in modern medicine can be treated by the following methods.

Applications of hand therapy:

1) Acupuncture therapy:

(1) At regular and extra acupoints:

Location: Neiguan (PC 6), Hegu (LI 4), Shangyang (LI 1) and Shaoshang (LU 11) acupoints.

Method of manipulation: Bleeding therapy is applied at Shangyang (LI 1) and Shaoshang (LU 11) acupoints; and the routine acupuncture is applied at Neiguan (PC 6) and Hegu (LI 4) with strong needling stimulation and retention of needles for 30 minutes.

(2) At reflective points:

Location: Throat point and tonsil point.

Method of manipulation: The needles are inserted for 1 cm and retained for five minutes.

2) Hand bath:

Recipe: Mabo (Fructus Lasiosphaera) 15 g, Shegan (Rhizoma Balamcandae) 15 g, Zisu (perilla leaf) 15 g, Pugongying (Herba Taraxaci) 30 g, Yinhua (Flos Lonicerae) 30 g, Niubangzi (burdock) 30 g, and Bohe (Herba Menthae) 6 g.

Function: To relieve toxicity and sore throat.

Method of manipulation: A hot decoction of these herbs is used to steam and wash both hands for 20 minutes, two to three times a day.

6. Sore throat

This is a disease of the throat with redness, swelling and pain.

Acute and chronic pharyngitis can be treated by the following methods.

Applications of hand therapy:

Acupuncture therapy:

At regular and extra acupoints.

Location: Hegu (LI 4), Shaoshang (LU 11) and Shangyang (LI 1) acupoints.

Method of manipulation: Bleeding therapy is applied at Shaoshang (LU 11) and Shangyang (LI 1), and the routine acupuncture is applied at Hegu (LI 4) with the needle retained for 30 minutes.

7. Deviation of mouth

This is a disease with deviation of mouth and eye.

Facial palsy in modern medicine can be treated by the following methods.

Applications of hand therapy:

1) Massage therapy:

Location: Head, mouth, eye, liver, and kidney areas, fingers, head acupoint beside the second metacarpal bone, Erjian (LI 2) and Hegu (LI 4) acupoints.

Method of manipulation: Pressing and kneading maneuvers applied to head, mouth, eye, liver, and kidney areas; digit-pressing and kneading maneuvers at Erjian (LI 2), Hegu (LI 4) and head acupoints; twisting, pulling, and rotating fingers.

2) Acupuncture therapy:

(1) At regular and extra acupoints:

Location: Hegu (LI 4) and Quchi (LI 11) acupoints.

Method of manipulation: The needles are retained for 30 minutes.

(2) At reflective areas:

Location: The corresponding areas of the face in the palmar reflective areas and ulnar or radial reverse palmar reflective areas.

Method of manipulation: The needles are shallowly inserted, but not retained.

3) Herb-holding therapy:

Herbs: Mahuang (Herba Ephedrae) 6 g, Fangji (Radix Stephaniae Tetrandrae) 6 g, Jingjie (Herba Schizonepetae) 6 g, Guizhi (cassia twig) 9 g, Chuanxiong (Rhizoma Ligustici) 15 g, Fangfeng (Radix Ledebouriellae) 2 g, and Fuzi (Aconite) 4 g.

Method of manipulation: A powder of these herbs is mixed with a paste of green onion stalks for holding in the palms to induce slight sweating, once a day.

8. Myopia

This is an eye condition with normal near sight but impaired far sight.

Myopia, axial myopia, indicia myopia and pseudomyopia in modern medicine are included under this condition and can be treated by the following methods.

Applications of hand therapy:

1) Massage therapy:

Location: Midline of palm, eye area, liver area, kidney area, Erjian (LI 2), Dagukong (EX-UE 5), Xiaogukong (EX-UE 6) and head area.

Method of manipulation: Rubbing midline of palm, digit-pressing and kneading maneuvers applied at eye, kidney and liver areas; digit-pressing and pinching maneuvers at Erjian (LI 2), Dagukong (EX-UE 5), Xiaogukong (EX-UE 6), and head area. The patient is asked to close his eyes, concentrate his attention on the eyeballs, and turn them from side to side.

2) Acupuncture therapy:

(1) At regular and extra acupoint:

Location: Hegu (LI 4) acupoint.

Method of manipulation: The needle is inserted and retained for 30 minutes.

(2) At reflective points:

Location: Eye point and liver point.

Method of manipulation: The needles are inserted for 1 cm and retained for five minutes after medium stimulation.

(3) At reflective areas:

Location: Eye area in palmar reflective areas and ulnar or radial reverse palmar reflective areas.

Method of manipulation: The needles are not retained.

9. Pseudomembranous conjunctivitis

This is an acute eye disease with apparent redness, swelling, hotness, and pain in the eyes caused by external wind and heat pathogens.

Pseudomembranous conjunctivitis is similar to this disease and can be treated by the following methods.

Applications of hand therapy:

1) Acupuncture therapy:

(1) At regular and extra acupoints:

Location: Guanchong (TE 1), Shangyang (LI 1) and Hegu (LI 4) acupoints.

Method of manipulation: Bleeding therapy is applied at Guanchong and Shangyang acupoints, and routine acupuncture is applied at Hegu with the needle retained for 30 minutes.

(2) At reflective points:

Location: Eye and liver points.

Method of manipulation: Bleeding therapy is applied at above points.

(3) At special acupoint beside the second metacarpal bone.

Location: Head acupoint.

Method of manipulation: Bleeding therapy is applied at above point.

2) Hand bath:

Recipe: Pugongying (Herba Taraxaci) 30 g, Juhua (chrysanthemum) 20 g, Kushen (Shrubby Sophora) 20 g and Xiakucao (Spica Prunellae) 20 g.

Function: To clear heat, relieve toxicity, clear liver heat, and improve vision.

Method of manipulation: A hot decoction of the above herbs is used to steam and wash both hands and eye region for 20 minutes, two to three times a day.

10. Scleritis

This is an eye disease with underlying and bulging swollen sclera tissue also scattered on the surface with localized purplish red nodules.

Scleritis in modern medicine is similar to this disease and can be treated by the methods mentioned for pseudomembranous conjunctivitis.

11. Paralytic strabismus

This is a sudden onset of eyeball deviation with limited eyeball movement and double vision.

Paralytic strabismus in modern medicine is similar and can be treated by the following methods.

Applications of hand therapy:

Acupuncture therapy:

(1) At regular and extra acupoints:

Location: Zhongdu (TE 3) and Hegu (LI 4) acupoints.

Method of manipulation: The needles are retained for 30 minutes after medium needling stimulation.

(2) At reflective points:

Location: Eye and liver points.

Method of manipulation: The needles are inserted for 1 cm and retained for five minutes.

12. Glaucoma

This is an eye disease with tense eyeball, dilated and greenish pupil, and marked impairment of vision which may cause blindness. It is often caused by emotional excitement or over fatigue, and in the early stages the patient may suffer from slight distension of eyeball, ipsilateral frontal headache, soreness of the nose, and blurred vision as though the eyeball were covered by fog. After a rest, the symptoms may disappear, but if not effectively treated serious clinical manifestations of glaucoma may appear. In traditional Chinese medicine glaucoma can be divided into two types: The prompt onset of greenish glaucoma and the insidious onset of bluish glaucoma.

Glaucoma in modern medicine is similar and can be treated by the following methods.

Applications of hand therapy:

1) Massage therapy:

Location: Palm, fingers, liver, kidney, and eye areas, Dagukong (EX-UE 5), Xiaogukong (EX-UE 6), Shangyang (LI 1), Shaoze (SI 1) and Houxi (SI 3) acupoints.

Method of manipulation: Pushing and pressing the palmar and both sides of fingers; pushing and grinding maneuvers applied to liver, eye, and kidney areas, Shangyang (LI 1), Shaoze (SI 1), and Houxi (SI 3) acupoints. During application of massage, the patient is asked to relax his body with eyes closed and concentrate attention on the eyes.

2) Acupuncture therapy:

(1) At regular and extra acupoint:

Location: Hegu (LI 4) acupoint.

Method of manipulation: The strong stimulation is applied and the needle is retained for 30 minutes.

(2) At reflective points:

Location: Eye and liver points.

Method of manipulation: The needles are retained for five minutes.

(3) At special acupoints beside the second metacarpal bone:

Location: Head acupoint and liver acupoint.

Method of manipulation: The needles are inserted for 1.6 cm

and retained for 15 minutes.

13. Optic nerve atrophy

This is an eye disease with progressive impairment of vision leading to complete blindness, although the appearance of the eyes is completely normal.

Optic nerve atrophy in modern medicine is similar and can be treated by the methods mentioned for glaucoma.

Applications of hand therapy:

As to acupuncture therapy, please refer to the methods of treating glaucoma.

14. Drooping upper eyelid

In patients with this disease the upper eyelids are drooped down and cannot be raised, so that the pupils are partially or completely covered, interfering with vision.

Ptosis of the upper eyelid in patients with myasthenia gravis can be treated by the following methods.

Applications of hand therapy:

Acupuncture therapy:

(1) At regular and extra acupoints:

Location: Hegu (LI 4) and Zhongdu (TE 3) acupoints.

Method of manipulation: The medium needling stimulation is applied and the needles are retained for 20 minutes.

(2) At reflective points:

Location: Eye point, spleen point, and liver point.

Method of manipulation: The needles are inserted for 1 cm and retained for five minutes after medium needling stimulation.

图书在版编目(CIP)数据

手疗治百病:英文/王胜,王卫东主编. 一北京:
外文出版社,1997(1998 重印)
(中医传统医疗实用小丛书)
ISBN 7 - 119 - 01901 - 5

Ⅰ.手… Ⅱ.①王… ②王… Ⅲ.手 - 外治法 -
英文 Ⅳ.R244.9

中国版本图书馆 CIP 数据核字 (97) 第 05028 号

责任编辑　孙海玉
插图绘制　李士伋

手疗治百病

王　胜　王卫东　主编

＊

©外文出版社
外文出版社出版
(中国北京百万庄大街 24 号)
邮政编码 100037
北京外文印刷厂印刷
中国国际图书贸易总公司发行
(中国北京车公庄西路 35 号)
北京邮政信箱第 399 号　邮政编码 100044
1997 年(大 32 开)第 1 版
1998 年第 1 版第 2 次印刷
(英)
ISBN 7 - 119 - 01901 - 5 /R·137(外)
03480
14 - E - 3119P